CW00847789

Star Throwers is a charit
supporting people affec
awareness and understaı
alternative/complementary  uvaume
information on new treatment options, including
clinical trials, to help patients make a well-informed
decision. Our complementary therapies and
counselling services are also available to help
patients and carers with the stress and difficulties of
coping with cancer in their lives.

Whether someone has been recently diagnosed, are
undergoing treatment, or have been told they have a
late-stage cancer and "there is nothing left that can
be done" for them, Star Throwers will provide
support every step of the way.

This book is designed to empower cancer patients by
providing credible and scientifically accurate
information to help them navigate a difficult and
complex journey.

Pan Pantziarka is a scientist, patient advocate and a
Trustee of Star Throwers. He combines deep
personal experience, professional knowledge and a
commitment to improving outcomes for cancer
patients. Making science accessible to all is
important – and this book aims to do just that.

*All proceeds from this book will be donated
to Star Throwers*

The Star Throwers Guide To Cancer

# The Star Throwers Guide To Cancer

Pan Pantziarka

*New Paradigm Publishing*

ISBN-13: 978-1537419251

ISBN-10: 1537419250

*For George and Gina, in loving memory.*

# Contents

# Acknowledgements

This book could not have been produced without the support of a generous grant to Star Throwers from Together Against Cancer – a charity dedicated to 'helping people with cancer through health education and empowering patients in helping them survive.' We hope that this book makes a contribution to those important and laudable aims.

Thanks are also due to everyone at Star Throwers – the staff, volunteers and patients and families. In particular, thanks to Henry, Tina, Steven, Neil, Janice and Rachel for support and input during the process of writing and publishing this book.

Finally, a big thank you to my wife, Irene Kappes, for her copy-editing and the numerous suggestions for improving the final version of the text.

The Star Throwers Guide To Cancer

# Foreword

A diagnosis of cancer comes as a shock to most people as we tend to think this is a disease that other people get, but not you or a close member of your family. The truth is almost everyone knows someone with cancer, but the average person's understanding of what is meant by cancer and, more importantly, the treatment options available, is minimal as people shy away from it due to fear.

Once cancer is diagnosed, the situation totally changes and it is only through knowledge and understanding of the disease that we can increase our chances of the best possible outcome.

Unlike many books, this one is based on personal experience. Pan Pantziarka lost his first wife, Gina, and then his son, George, to this disease. In the quest to find a cure for his son he learned how the medical system works not only here in the UK but also in other parts of the world. Through years of experience he learned how to interact with oncologists and other members of the medical profession, which is knowledge that can never be valued highly enough.

In addition, as a mathematical modeller and a scientist, his reasoning is solid and one can be assured that all the advice in this book is based on years of research and study, as well as direct personal experience.

If you want one book full of excellent practical advice and understanding, for anyone suffering from cancer, then this is it. I would not hesitate to say that you will learn more from this book than any other I have come across. It will arm you with the knowledge to get the best out of the system and as a result increase your chances of the best possible outcome.

Dr Henry Mannings

*Founder of Star Throwers*

# Introduction

## What makes a good guidebook?

Welcome to the *Star Throwers Guide To Cancer* –
which we have billed as an 'in-depth guide for
patients'. Our intention in producing this book is to
provide cancer patients and carers with a useful
guide that can help them in the complex journey that
follows a cancer diagnosis. So, to all intents and
purposes this is a guidebook, just like any other.
Now guidebooks come in all shapes and sizes, from
those designed to outline the most well-trodden
tourist routes to those that specialise in out of the
way places that are way off the beaten track. Some
guidebooks will be light on detail and not much use
if you stray from the path, while others are designed
only for the most intrepid travellers and are filled
with dense layers of detail.

As with travelling, a similar situation exists when it
comes to cancer guidebooks. There are plenty of
books on cancer currently available, many of them
specifically designed to help patients dealing with
the disease and treatment. Many of these will cover
the basics – going over well-known paths and being
light on detail. If you have to stray from those paths
for whatever reason then you're stuck and left

without a map to help you navigate unfamiliar territory. We hope that this book is different – this is a book explicitly designed to give you a compass, some landmarks and the tools you need to find the destinations that you want to find.

In practice this means providing the reader with scientifically-grounded information on:

- Understanding clinical trials and where and how to search for them
- How to search for and access treatments abroad
- Stress and cancer, including a range of practical techniques to reduce stress
- How to do your own research, including making sense of academic papers and clinical trial results
- Understanding how to interpret cancer-related stories in the mass media, including so-called 'miracle cures'
- Different forms of treatment, including tumour ablation treatments such as cryoablation, photodynamic therapy and radiofrequency ablation

Just this sample of the topics covered in the book should indicate that this is not designed to be a simplistic retelling of the basic information published by other cancer charities and medical authorities, much of it available via the internet.

While that information is essential and important, it is assumed that the readers of this book are looking for something with more depth and more immediately geared towards seeking new treatment options or a greater understanding of cancer treatments.

If there's a theme that underlies this whole project it's the simple one of empowering patients as much as possible. This means providing both the information and intellectual tools necessary to engage with the medical literature and, just as importantly, with clinicians on a more equal footing. The latter is actually not an easy task – in fact it's one that many patients feel they can never do. It's crazy if you think about it – when faced with a life-threatening diagnosis there are still too many patients afraid to question decisions or even engage in an honest discussion. There are also many doctors who are still stuck with the idea that patients should be passive consumers of medical treatment and, if we are honest, there are just as many patients who want to leave it to the experts to decide on their behalf. Unfortunately, cancer is far too complex a disease, and far too serious a health issue, for such a simplistic relationship to work, particularly if initial treatments start to fail.

So, one of the aims of this book is to change that doctor-patient relationship – both by suggesting specific strategies to handle the relationship, and by providing advice on where to find useful high quality information rather than relying on newspaper headlines or dubious content on the internet.

## The Star Throwers Ethos

In addition to wanting to inform patients who are looking for new treatment options, or who simply want to learn more about their disease or medical research, this book is also designed to reflect the ethos of Star Throwers. To quote from the Star Throwers website:

*We believe cancer sufferers and their families deserve compassionate care, guidance and support at any stage of their cancer - whether they have just received a cancer diagnosis, are trying to understand the diagnosis and its implications, are deciding between treatment options, managing treatment related side effects, or needing support with post-treatment cancer survivorship.*

*We specialise in supporting cancer sufferers that have been diagnosed as 'terminal' and have been offered no treatments other than palliative care. Many patients feel they are not ready to accept that nothing further can be done to help them and would like to explore all the options available to them. Our approach is to provide compassionate guidance and support with the goal of maximizing both quantity and quality of life.*

The many cancer patients, and their families and friends, who have visited Star Throwers know that these are not empty phrases or lofty aspirations. I know from my own personal experience that Dr Henry Mannings is one of the most dedicated and humane doctors I have ever met. I know too that Henry is supported by an experienced and dedicated team and that together they make Star Throwers the unique place that it is. There are many cancer support charities and centres, but Star Throwers is different.

Partly this is down to a simple philosophy that says it is up to patients to decide when they want to stop exploring treatment options. Where some physicians will work with patients who want to look at additional options once the standard treatments have failed, there are also many who do not have the time or inclination and are content instead to transfer patients to palliative care. Star Throwers will work with people to see what else can be done. Often this means searching for clinical trials. But it may also mean looking at different treatment scenarios, for example the use of *metronomic* chemotherapy or the use of *repurposed drugs* (and there are chapters on both these topics later in the book).

A key point about this important avenue of support is that it is scientifically grounded. Unfortunately there is no shortage of people out there who claim to have 'cures' or 'break-through treatments'. Some of these people are simply crooks out to fleece desperate cancer patients with high-priced 'treatments' that provide no real benefit. In some cases these so-called treatments can actually do harm and they nearly always create vast profits for the people peddling them. In other cases people are simply repeating unfounded claims about treatments because they are genuine believers and have the best of motives. In either case however the risks are real.

While critical of some doctors and some aspects of current medical practice, the Star Throwers approach is one of honest scepticism rather than one that rejects science and scientific thinking. The same approach has been adopted in this book. For example in the chapter on 'Cancer and the Media' there is a lot of discussion on ways to detect scams and spot the 'conspiracy theories' used to convince people that there are cancer cures that have been suppressed in order to benefit the drugs companies and doctors. This approach is always about looking for evidence

– whether it's an alternative or complementary treatment or some new drug from a pharma company, the question has to come down to evidence. When dealing with advanced disease, with no standard treatments on offer, the standard of evidence that is acceptable may be very different to early stage disease with a good prognosis. In the latter case you want evidence from large Phase III clinical trials, but when a patient is told there are no standard treatments on offer, the level of evidence will often be more speculative. But even in that case *evidence is required* – in contrast to those people selling untested 'miracle cures' on the internet.

Another important point to make is that there is no hidden agenda at work. The staff at Star Throwers are not out to sell a product, philosophy or lifestyle. Where there are some support groups and organisations which have a very distinct narrative – that cancer is due to environmental toxins, dairy produce, sugar in the diet or that it can be treated using specific products, diets or lifestyle changes – there is no one at Star Throwers trying to 'sell' anything. It is, essentially, a very independent and pragmatic approach that puts the needs of the person being supported centre stage.

## About the author

Finally, a few words about the author of this book: Pan Pantziarka.

If we return again to the guidebook analogy – key questions to ask about the person writing it are: What are his or her qualifications? How well does he or she know the territory? The best way to answer those questions is by telling you a little bit about myself, my connections to Star Throwers and my experiences with cancer.

I work as a scientist for a Belgian charity called the Anticancer Fund, primarily involved in drug repurposing research (this is about looking at the use of existing non-cancer drugs as new cancer treatments, a topic covered more fully in a separate chapter). I have also published research on the rare genetic cancer condition called Li Fraumeni Syndrome – and this is where my personal and professional lives collide.

By training I am an engineer with a PhD in computer science, but for much of my working life I was what is now frequently called a 'data scientist' – this is the combination of software, statistics and analysis that is fast becoming a separate academic discipline. My introduction to the reality of cancer came in 1994 when my first wife, Gina, was diagnosed with ovarian cancer. She was 29 years old at the time and had been feeling run down following the birth of our son, our second child, 14 months previously. The diagnosis came as a shock; it was the last thing either of us had expected. By then the disease was already very advanced – her body was riddled with metastases and she was seriously ill. She died before we had even come to terms with what was happening – she lost consciousness a few days after the diagnosis and within three weeks she was gone.

At the time I knew next to nothing about cancer. Even now, many years later, I can vividly remember the fear, confusion and distress that the diagnosis brought with it.

Ten months later, my son George developed a hard lump on the left side of his face. It took a number of visits to doctors and hospitals before we finally found out that it too was a cancer. It was a rhabdomyosarcoma in his left temporalis muscle, and we received the diagnosis on his second birthday at Great Ormond Street Hospital. At the time I felt that this had to be connected to his mother's cancer, but we were assured that there was no connection between ovarian cancer and sarcoma.

George was treated with chemotherapy and surgery and, after completing the gruelling treatment, he was declared in remission. It had been tough but we hoped that it was behind us and that we could look forward to starting our lives again. Somehow George had managed to remain a happy and energetic child with a lust for life that was phenomenal. A few months later we noticed a swelling where the tumour had been. Again I was told that I was being a paranoid parent but a few weeks later the swelling was unmistakable and the disease had recurred. This time George was treated with second line chemo, surgery and radiotherapy.

At the end of the treatment, the final pathology showed evidence of residual disease. He was still the lively and boisterous kid that he had always been, but the prognosis was clear. In no uncertain terms we were told that we had to prepare for the worst – there were no more chemo drugs, no more radiotherapy and surgery was not going to work. There was, we were told, less than a 5% chance of survival. We refused to accept this – how could we? By this time I had been reading everything I could on cancer, including alternative treatments and experimental therapies.

We asked for a second opinion and transferred George's care to the Royal Marsden. We started giving George different vitamins, Chinese herbs, we played visualisation games where he fought the 'bad stuff', we changed diet… And all the time we waited for the disease to come back. But although there were a few scares along the way, including a suspicious growth in his ear which turned out to be benign, there was no sign of the rhabdomyosarcoma.

Fast forward to George at fifteen: a fit, healthy and active teenager obsessed with computer games and hanging out with his friends at school. He was fine apart from some slight facial disfigurements from his various surgeries and treatments. A routine visit to the GP uncovered a dark patch on his scalp, just behind the ear. It turned out to be a second cancer – a basal cell carcinoma that was surgically excised almost as soon as it was discovered. But the fear was back and the shock of the diagnosis jolted all of us.

And then, just a few weeks later, his upper lip started to tingle, and his jaw started to ache. He was fairly relaxed about it all but the rest of the family were frantic with worry. Eventually a CT scan revealed something nasty in his jaw. A biopsy told us that this was a bone cancer – an osteosarcoma. This made three different cancers before the age of sixteen – which finally prompted a gene test. It revealed that he had the rare genetic condition called Li Fraumeni Syndrome which is caused by a mutation in the TP53 tumour suppressor gene – the body's main line of defence against cells turning cancerous – a genetic condition which we now presume he had inherited from his mother.

By this time I was armed with a PhD and had access to university libraries. While George underwent chemo and surgery, (including having half his jaw removed and replaced with a rib and then again with his fibula), I was reading and researching and contacting doctors and scientists all over the world as the standard treatments started to fail. When the standard treatments ended he had photodynamic therapy in London, chemo-perfusion in Frankfurt, cryoablation and immunotherapy in China.

In the process of seeking different options I made contact with Star Throwers and Dr Henry Mannings. We discussed the option of a form of immunotherapy called Coley's Toxins, which had been developed in the late nineteenth century by a surgeon who used it to treat bone cancers. Dr Mannings applied to the MHRA to import the treatment so that it could be used on George, but it took so long to get approval that the disease was very advanced by the time we got the go ahead. But despite the late stage George wanted to go ahead and give it a try – he wanted to live and there were few options left.

Sadly it was already too late and George passed away on 25<sup>th</sup> April 2011.

Later George's stepmum and I formed the George Pantziarka TP53 Trust to support other families suffering from the same genetic condition. I was also asked to become a Trustee at Star Throwers, which I accepted. And in 2013 I published my first scientific paper on cancer, a paper on Li Fraumeni Syndrome. Since then I have moved full-time from data science to oncology, and continue to publish research papers on Li Fraumeni Syndrome and on drug repurposing.

I have described these personal events to make plain that I have faced many of the dilemmas that cancer patients have to face. I have had to search for treatment options, argue with doctors, seek treatments abroad, assess evidence and get to grips with the many topics discussed in this book.

Most importantly I have endeavoured to write the book that I wish I had had available to me when going through some of the tough times I described above. I hope that I've managed to do that and that this is a useful guide in your own cancer journey.

Pan Pantziarka

May 2016

# You and Your Treatment

## Introduction

There are few experiences more frightening and disorientating than being diagnosed with cancer. The diagnosis, when it finally comes, is likely to have been preceded by a period of increasing concern, multiple visits to doctors and hospitals, a battery of diagnostic tests and imaging. In many cases the diagnosis is merely a confirmation of the fact that has become apparent to all during the diagnostic process. Regardless of whether the diagnosis is for you, a partner, a child or other loved one, the period running up to it has probably been extremely stressful and trying. And, once the diagnosis has been received, there is hardly time to catch breath before treatment plans have to be discussed, decisions made and treatments begun. This chapter looks at some of the practical issues related to being a cancer patient or carer rather than focusing on science or treatments as the other chapters will do. Nevertheless it will discuss important issues that need to be addressed, such as the relationship with your doctor, practical issues relating to appointments and how to deal with concerned relatives and friends.

Obviously there are readers who are at different stages of their cancer journey, some may still be in the process of being diagnosed, others may already be in treatment and some may be in second or third line treatments. As this chapter will attempt to cover issues at all stages, from the initial period to much later, there may be some material which will not be applicable to you. This chapter also assumes that the reader is the patient, although the content will also be relevant to carers and those, like parents of children with cancer, who have to help make decisions about treatment options.

No matter who the reader is, this chapter is about adjusting to the difficult and stressful life of a cancer patient. For newly diagnosed patients, in addition to the shock, there is a feeling of loss of control in the face of a complex new world that operates on different time scales, with a new language to learn, new rules of engagement and little time or space to adjust. The aim of this chapter then, is to help in the process of adjusting and in taking back some measure of control during one of the most difficult journeys you have to make.

## What Is An Oncologist?

Simply put an oncologist is a doctor who specialises in the treatment of cancer. This is actually a very broad definition because there are in fact many different types of doctors who treat cancer, with different specialisms in terms of the cancers they treat and the methods that they use. Generally when people talk of oncologists they are thinking of medical oncologists, who are the doctors who treat cancers using chemotherapy, hormonal treatments and other drugs. However, there are also surgical oncologists, who very obviously treat cancer using surgery, and radiation oncologists who use radiotherapy and different forms of ablation treatments (see the chapter on Ablative Therapies for more details on these). Most cancer treatments actually involve more than one form of therapy (often referred to as a treatment *modality*), for example chemotherapy and radiotherapy in combination, and it is usually the medical oncologist who is the main consultant in overall charge. In this document the term oncologist is in line with common usage and means the medical oncologist unless stated otherwise.

Oncologists come in all shapes and sizes and have very different personalities, just like the rest of us, but overall they are pessimists based on the reality that, despite their best efforts, successful treatment is not a common enough outcome, although it does occur. While the cancer experience is new and terrifying to you, they will have seen people in your situation many times in the past. Inevitably this previous experience will colour their outlook, just as it would for us if the roles were reversed.

It's highly unlikely that you have had much say in the choice of oncologist. For most of us – patients, parents or carers – we will have had no chance to think about who we'd like to choose, things are too frantic and scary for much deliberation. If you have yet to meet your oncologist it is perhaps worth taking a moment before your first meeting to think about what you would ideally want from him or her.

Many questions may come to mind. For example, you may want to know how many years of experience they have in oncology. Or you may want to know how long they've been in their present position. Most oncologists specialise in two or three types of cancer. It is important to know how much interest they have in your specific type. For example, are they involved in research in your form of cancer? If so they may be more knowledgeable and be more aware of trials that you could enter if the need arises later. This is particularly important if you have one of the rarer cancers; in such situations it is important to ask how often they have treated people with your form of the disease.

Believe it or not it will be OK to ask these questions when you first meet your oncologist. Why? Because you need to build a relationship with this doctor that may last for many months or even years. You will have to place enormous amounts of trust in what they do, so asking some awkward questions is important from two perspectives. First because you want to know the answers, but possibly more importantly you will want to see how they react to the questions. If you get an affronted response and your questions are treated as insulting or impertinent then that doesn't bode well for creating a solid relationship built on trust. On the other hand, if the questions are answered honestly and without much fuss then that's a much more positive start.

And the content of those answers matters too, of course. However, it's not always possible to work out the true value of an answer. Partly this is down to how well you ask the questions. For example, asking a question about how often they treat cancer is not as good as asking the question about how often they treat *your* type of cancer, and even that's not as good as asking how often they've treated the specific sub-type of cancer that you've been diagnosed with.

Even more difficult to interpret is the question on research. On the face of it having an oncologist who has a great research record and is much in demand for conferences and lectures would seem a great idea. What can be better than being treated by a world class expert? The down-sides can be that your oncologist is so busy in the lab, in the conference hall or lecture theatre that they are not readily available to you, and may often have to skip clinic or delegate to more junior colleagues. Ideally you want an oncologist who is involved to some extent in research, particularly in clinical trials, but who is not more of a researcher than a clinician.

The main thing though is that you work on establishing a degree of trust early in the process. This is important because there may come a time when there is a need for some difficult discussions and you need to be able to have a frank conversation without feeling that you are stepping out of line. We should not underestimate how difficult it is to do this. On the whole we are still brought up to treat doctors with a deference and a respect that we give to few other professions. For a patient it can be enormously difficult to argue or disagree with their doctor, even when it is the case that the doctor would not be insulted or defensive in response. It makes sense, then, to work at establishing an open and honest relationship at the very beginning. And, although this may seem radical to some, it may be the case that if that relationship does not emerge quickly it would be better to seek a different oncologist earlier rather than later.

The simplest way to change consultant in the NHS is to ask for a second opinion. You can do this be asking your existing consultant, but if this is difficult or you feel uncomfortable then you can go back to your GP and ask for a new referral. The new consultant will be informed that you're seeking a second opinion and they will be granted access to your existing scan and biopsy results. The new consultant is not obliged to take on your case, but in general doctors will work with each other to accommodate a patient's wishes.

Finally, get your oncologist's email address. Ask for it outright, or else go on the hospital web site and get it there if it is available. There will be times when you want to ask a quick question, or want to discuss something you've read (for example about a new drug or treatment) at the next appointment. Being able to communicate outside of appointments, or to share articles in advance of a meeting, is important. If you just turn up at an appointment with an article for your doctor, then the chances are that it won't be read and discussed. Time is limited, and your doctor will be unable to read and respond given the time available. Send the article before the appointment and you have more chance of getting it discussed. Some doctors will be more than happy to communicate via email, while some will be a bit shocked. At worst your emails will be ignored, but at best you can engage in a dialogue that enables you to access support outside of a clinic or a hospital ward.

## Your First Oncology Appointment

This section is for those patients who have only just been referred to an oncologist and have yet to meet him or her. Generally, it is a physician or surgeon who, following a series of investigations, informs you that you have cancer. If it is a surgeon you may be offered surgery to remove the tumour if it is operable, but even in these cases you will normally also be referred to an oncologist to manage the additional treatments, usually chemotherapy, that are often included as part of a treatment protocol. Doctors are not generally good at breaking bad news and many will prefer to leave it to the oncologist to discuss the particular prognosis.

On your first meeting with your oncologist you'll normally find him or her accompanied by an oncology nurse and possibly one or more other doctors. At this moment you are probably having palpitations, having absolutely no idea what to expect. You have been told that you have cancer but have no real understanding of what this means. In your head, cancer means death and you may feel totally panicked as you are not ready to die.

Some oncologists will be very welcoming and stand up and shake your hand, giving an empathic smile that suggests they have a human and approachable side to them. Others will adopt a more formal approach, which they see as more professional, and act as though they are the expert and you are the patient who will unquestioningly do as you are told. This may seem cold and impersonal, but doctors have to place some emotional barriers between themselves and their patients if only to safe-guard their own psychological well-being. For others being in control is not just a defence mechanism but a key part of their professional personality.

Many people experience feelings of fear and panic, which are completely normal and expected, but it can be overwhelming. It does mean that in this situation, it's more difficult to take in or comprehend the information that will be supplied to you. Therefore it is imperative that you bring at least one other person with you for this appointment, preferably someone who is clear headed. The obvious person to bring with you is your partner, close family member or best friend – though beware that having someone with you who is even more freaked out than you are will not be helpful to anyone, least of all you. Possibly if you have a friend or family member who has a medical, nursing or scientific background, ask them to attend the appointment as well.

Often the oncologist will start by summarising the findings of the tests you have undergone and give you a formal diagnosis. This tells you how the various results have been analysed and assessed by the various doctors and teams you have seen so far, including the results of any biopsies (analysis of a sample of the tumour or suspicious lump), CT and MRI scans and other tests. The diagnosis will normally include a specific 'staging' – this is a measure of how far the disease has spread. This is all about where you are, but the big issue of course is the prognosis – the likely course of the disease and how treatment can influence that.

In terms of outlining your prognosis, the oncologist will tell you the recommended treatment for your cancer. This could be a hormone therapy, chemotherapy, radiotherapy or a combination of these depending on the type of tumour. Typically you will be presented with an outline of a protocol which will cover:

- which drugs are included – typically treatment will include multiple chemotherapy drugs to reduce the risks of disease resistance
- how many treatment cycles are required (in other words how many courses of treatment are needed) and what each cycle consists of
- the sequence of treatments – for example three cycles of chemotherapy and then radiotherapy followed by another two cycles of chemotherapy
- some idea of a time-line for your treatment – often this is discussed in terms of the number of weeks between the start and end of treatment
- time points for scanning or other imaging – this is to assess treatment response and possible re-staging depending on that response

If surgery is still an option then treatment with chemotherapy may be given either before surgery (neo-adjuvant) to reduce the size of the tumour or after surgery (adjuvant) to mop up any tumour cells that 'got away'. Common side-effects associated with the treatment, both minor and major, will also be discussed.

If you have had a chance to think about the kind of questions outlined in the previous section then now is the time to start asking them. Remember, just as you are trying to digest all this information and to gauge the oncologist, he or she is trying to gauge you in turn. It is also important to ask if the therapy is being given with curative or palliative intent, although unfortunately for some it will be the latter. In addition to the side effects of chemotherapy and radiotherapy, it is important to confirm that the stated improvements in survival are from the medical literature, as sometimes these benefits can be overstated by some oncologists.

In some cases you may also be offered the option of taking part in a clinical trial. If this is the case then you are advised to refer to the chapters on clinical trials, where you will find more details on what the different types of trial are and information which may help you to decide on whether to proceed with a trial or not.

At this stage, try to take in as much information as possible but do not make any decision. These are among the most important decisions you will ever have to make, so taking some time to digest the information calmly is the most sensible thing to do. The only exceptions to this are the rare situations where any delay could lead to death, such as in some leukaemias where a low platelet count could lead to severe haemorrhage.

Some people feel the need to ask the oncologist how long they have to live as they want to put their affairs in order or plan for the future of their families. Often if the patient does not ask, then this information will not be volunteered, so don't feel that you have to ask if you don't want to know. In any case the answer to the question will be given based on survival figures that compare survival for people with and without treatment. This survival figure is based on the statistics for a large group of patients and the most important thing to remember is that you are not a statistic, so this survival figure will probably not be based on the specifics of your particular case.

Most oncologists will appreciate that you need time to get your thoughts together and make a decision and will be happy for you to ring them with your decision on whether to proceed with the treatment they have outlined or not. In the meantime, you have to do your homework and research the treatment that has been offered. Please remember to make notes, or better still ask one of the people with you to make notes. See also the next section on preparing for appointments for advice on this.

If you have been told that your disease is incurable because your cancer is not amenable to surgery (not resectable is how it may be described by your doctor) then it is important to make certain that this really is the case. If the tumour has spread to other organs, then the reality is that surgery is not an option, although occasionally this can change later if the tumour turns out to be exceptionally responsive to chemotherapy. If there is no evidence of spread or distant disease then you have to ask why surgery is not an option. This sort of decision has to come from a surgeon, *not* from an oncologist or radiologist.

Some tumours are localised with no evidence of spread but are deemed inoperable because the tumour has encased vital blood vessels. In this situation it is imperative to get a second surgical opinion from a hospital that is known for performing surgery in that region of the body. Again, do not rely on a referral to a second oncologist as they have insufficient knowledge of the surgical skills required. Instead do some research on the internet to find a surgeon with a national or international reputation, and insist that you are referred to him or her.

Once a treatment plan has been agreed you will be given a treatment protocol that maps your treatment. It will have details of times and dates – for drugs, radiotherapy, surgery and the various scans and tests required to monitor how you are doing. There will be check-points where you will be 'restaged' and the plans changed depending on whether your disease is stable, increasing or decreasing.

## Preparing for Future Appointments

Meeting doctors will become a regular event, but when you are having different forms of treatment it's the major meetings with your oncologist that will assume the greatest importance, particularly when waiting for results from scans or examinations. Some patients term the anxious wait for scan results 'scanxiety', for obvious and understandable reasons.

At times like this you will be stressed and apprehensive. No matter how much you like or respect your doctors, you'll be feeling tense and nervous. Sitting in the waiting room can be hard, especially if the clinic is running late and you've been waiting for ages. At times like these it's easy to get so stressed that you forget to ask the things you've been meaning to ask. It's ridiculous, because you may have been waiting for ages to ask these questions, but you can be blindsided by news (good or bad), get diverted by some other train of thought or simply forget everything and just sit there passively while the doctor leads the discussion.

Afterwards, you'll kick yourself for not having remembered to ask your questions and will either have to wait for the next appointment or get on the phone or look for someone else to ask.

So, the first rule for seeing your doctor, particularly for those big meetings to discuss scan results or re-staging, is to prepare in advance. First and foremost, take the time to sit down and go through what it is you want to know. Don't leave it to the last minute if you can. Write down your questions, discuss them with family or friends if necessary, but make sure you have them on paper. Writing the questions down might seem such a pointless thing to do, but it will pay dividends in keeping focused and making sure that you get the information that you need, not just the information the doctor thinks you need.

Having your questions in front of you also has a fringe benefit in that you have pen and paper to hand. If your oncologist mentions a drug, treatment or side effect that you've never heard of before then write it down. There's nothing more infuriating then coming away from a meeting and only half remembering important details. And a lot of the drugs that are used in oncology have weird names (bevacizumab, imatinib etc) that are hard to remember clearly – you need them written down. Don't be afraid to stop and ask for the spelling. The drugs may just trip off the tongue of a specialist, but for patients they are all new and strange sounding. It's the same for treatments – intra-arterial chemoembolisation, photodynamic therapy and so on are hard to remember, especially if you've just received bad news.

Keeping pen and paper to hand is useful to get a note of all these. And tick off the questions that are answered so that you can make sure that nothing is missed. Take the time to look at your list, especially if the meeting is a difficult one. At the end of the appointment if anything has been missed, then go back to it. It takes a certain amount of discipline to do this, and you may be a bit nervous about appearing odd, but it's more important that you get the information you need. Unfortunately, it is often still true that the default position in many clinics is for the patient to be a passive receiver of treatment, who is not expected to ask questions or be difficult. That might be fine if you're dealing with a bit of an infection, but when you're dealing with a disease like cancer you need to take more control. And, believe it or not, you'll feel better for having that degree of control.

Meetings about re-staging are especially important and therefore often tense. Sometimes the oncologist will tell you how effective the treatment has been in terms of response. This is described as a 'complete' or 'partial response' but it is imperative you understand what is meant by this as it can be easily misinterpreted. A complete response means that the tumour has disappeared on a CT or MRI scan or that tumour markers in the bloodstream have normalised. A partial response means that the tumour has shrunk by at least 50%, if it has shrunk less than 50% it is classified as 'stable disease'. If the tumour has continued to grow, the oncologist refers to this as 'progressive disease'.

The best response is described as a 'complete response', which means that there is no evidence of tumour at that time. This is obviously good news and something that we want to maintain permanently. However, strictly speaking a complete response just means that there is no evidence of a tumour for a period of a few weeks, sometimes even for only a month. In many cases there are microscopic pockets of disease left behind and these may start growing again and turn into recurrent or relapsed disease. So, if you do have chemotherapy and are told that you have had a complete response to the treatment it does not mean you are cured. In reality the tumour could be back in a few weeks or months. It simply means that you are currently in a state where there is no disease apparent and are therefore classified as having a complete response.

## Lines of Communication

So far in this chapter we have focused on the relationship between patient and doctor and how to strive to build a relationship that works. But it is not the only area where communications are likely to be difficult at times. For example other important relationships may also be strained at time, for example with a partner, close family and friends and so on. A recent study that looked at this found that 'managing communication around cancer diagnosis gives patients a sense of control in an otherwise uncontrollable situation' [1]. The researchers found that:

*...communication is an important factor in coping with cancer in that it enables people to exert control during a highly stressful and turbulent time. However, despite best efforts to structure and control that communication, cancer patients cannot always predict or control other people's reaction.*

The need to communicate with friends and family can simply became exhausting, particularly when you've just had bad news. The need to relay it multiple times just makes you feel worse. The constant repetition of bad news is depressing, especially when you know that the person on the other end is going to react badly to it too. It means that not only do you have to deal with your own reactions, but you end up having to manage other people too. It increases the stress precisely when you're most stressed out.

Of course the person on the other end of the line isn't deliberately adding to the pressure. They are concerned and mostly want to help in some way, possibly by giving you a shoulder to cry on. What they often don't realise is that they are not the only people calling, and that sometimes you need the space to think and absorb news (good or bad). Receiving a concerned phone call as soon as you've had a difficult meeting with your oncologist or other doctor is especially exhausting. When you're uncertain how to feel after receiving scan results, or a new disease staging or diagnosis, having to relay the news is simply hard to do.

In the end one way to solve the problem, at least to a certain extent, is by nominating one or two people as the key points of contact and communicating with everyone else through them. That way you can impose some control over the situation. It means that you have time and space to absorb news, to think about things, to focus your energies where you need them focused. When you have something to report you just relay it once or twice and then let the news filter out to the wider community of friends and family without you being directly involved unless you want to be.

An alternative approach is to use a blog, Facebook or other social network to communicate to friends and family alike. Not only is this a good way to issue updates, it's also a good way to get support and advice. This is particularly the case when you can become part of an online community of people going through the same thing – for example online support groups for breast cancer or people undergoing the same treatment.

## Seeking Help

Finally, it is important to mention that while this cancer journey is new to you and your family, there are lots of other people going through the same journey and coming up against the same issues. Fortunately there are many ways to gain additional support and advice, from national organisations like Macmillan Cancer Support or CLIC Sargent, to local support organisations like Star Throwers to online forums and patient-support groups specific to different cancers. The support is out there to be accessed – there is no need to suffer loneliness and isolation in addition to the rigours of being a cancer patient or a carer. It is not weakness to seek support, especially at a difficult time like this.

## Summary

- Although many doctors will be involved in treating a cancer patient, it is normally a medical oncologist who has overall charge – it is important to build a positive relationship with your oncologist
- Much of the language of oncology is complex and unfamiliar
- Prepare for appointments in advance, particularly those appointments around results and restaging – make a list of questions and be ready to take notes (always have pen and paper with you!)
- Having to relay your news to multiple family members and friends can be emotionally draining – you can lessen this by nominating a trusted person as your 'line of communication' who can pass on information to a wider set of people

## References

1       Donovan-Kicken E, Tollison AC and Goins ES (2011) **A Grounded Theory of Control**

over **Communication Among Individuals with Cancer**. *Journal of Applied Communication Research*, **39**(3), pp. 310–330.

# Stress and Cancer

## Introduction

Having cancer is stressful – both physically and emotionally. In many cases the stress begins even before the formal diagnosis is delivered – and it only gets worse once treatment begins in earnest. This chapter will look at some of the evidence for the impacts that stress has on cancer, evidence which shows that excessive stress can actually act to enhance tumour growth. However, there is also evidence to show that acting to reduce that stress can have very positive effects, including evidence that it may impact overall survival and reduce the risks of disease recurrence.

Furthermore, this chapter will explore a range of interventions which have been shown to reduce stress levels in cancer. This chapter is intended to help *you* manage stress, and is therefore useful not only for cancer patients but also for friends and family.

## What is Stress?

What we know as stress is actually part of the 'fight or flight' syndrome that is essential for survival – it is the response which functions at a largely unconscious level to help us deal with situations which require an immediate reaction. While it may have evolved when our ancestors had to worry about becoming lunch for large predators, or victim to a raiding party from a neighbouring clan, these days it's what causes drivers to swerve to avoid hitting someone who's stepped into the road without looking. The responses are instant, often before we have even consciously registered that there's danger ahead. The threats that we respond to can be real or imagined but once a threat has registered everything else that follows is automatic.

This 'fight or flight' response is fast acting and depends on the release of chemical messages (hormones) that trigger a cascade of physiological responses: increased heart rate, hyper-alertness, shallower breathing, increase of blood glucose levels and so on. This acute response is triggered in part by the release of a class of hormones called catecholamines, which includes epinephrine and norepinephrine (more commonly known in the UK as adrenaline and noradrenaline), which set in train these physical responses. They also trigger the release of other chemical messages that lead to further changes. At the same time there are feedback loops which cut off these physical responses once the danger has passed. The system is finely tuned and has evolved as a transient response to maximise your chance of survival to a specific threat. We can see then that this acute stress response is a vital and necessary part of life.

However, in this context we are talking not about an acute stress response but *chronic stress* – in other words activation of some elements of the 'fight or flight' syndrome on an ongoing basis in response to threats or dangers that are not easily or quickly resolved. Chronic stress can be brought on by external or environmental circumstances – for example living in over-crowded conditions, coping with noisy neighbours or losing your job – and also by psychological or emotional factors such as worrying about the future, dealing with a difficult relationship and so on. Where acute stress is essential and beneficial, the effects of chronic stress are not.

Physiologically chronic stress is associated with elevated release of stress hormones (including epinephrine, norepinephrine and cortisol), increased blood pressure, increased heart rate, a depressed immune system, digestive problems, increased fatigue etc. The psychological impacts of chronic stress include increased anxiety, insomnia, lack of concentration and depression. Of course physiology and psychology are linked – there is a feedback loop in which the physical symptoms of stress make the emotional response worse, and the worse feelings exacerbate the physical.

## Chronic Stress and Cancer

It is inevitable that a cancer diagnosis, or the fact of having to support a loved one with cancer, is stressful. Quite rightly we perceive this as a threat and of course we respond by becoming stressed. It is also clear that cancer is a threat that does not easily resolve and therefore often leads to chronic stress. It is also the case that many patients who have gone through treatment and have come out the other side and are in remission are still anxious, stressed and possibly depressed. All of this is quite natural and should not be anything that people should feel apologetic or guilty about. The question we need to address is whether this chronic stress has physical effects related to cancer.

The relationship between chronic stress and cancer is a complex one, with much that we still don't understand about it. Aside from everything else, there is a huge part of how we deal with stress that is down to individual personality and history – different people will react very differently to the same stressors. There is also the issue of stress preceding a cancer diagnosis – and in fact it is not uncommon for cancer patients to identify very stressful incidents prior to a cancer diagnosis and to then apportion part of the 'blame' for the cancer on that stress. Trying to make sense of all of this is no mean feat but in 2008 a group from University College London published a paper in the journal Nature Reviews Clinical Oncology entitled 'Do stress-related psychosocial factors contribute to cancer incidence and survival?' [1] This was a *meta-analysis*, (in which they put the data from different clinical trials together and then analyse it as a whole), designed to see if they could identify any relationships between stressful life events and the risks of developing or dying of cancer. It is a good starting point for exploring the issues in more depth.

The most important results from this meta-analysis were summarised as follows:

- Combined effects from large numbers of studies suggest that stress-related psychosocial factors have an adverse effect on cancer incidence, prognosis, and mortality – although the presence of *publication bias* means that these results should be interpreted with caution. [Note that publication bias happens when only those studies which show an association get published, a study which shows no relationship might not be considered interesting enough to get published – hence the possibility of bias in the data]

- Stressful life experiences were related to decreased cancer survival and increased mortality
- Stress-prone personality or unfavourable coping styles and emotional distress or poor quality of life were related to increased cancer incidence, reduced cancer survival and increased cancer mortality; in particular, depression seemed to be the primary driver of adverse effects of emotional distress

In addition to this meta-analysis there have been subsequent studies which have confirmed many of these findings, particularly with respect to the negative impacts of depression.

That was the bad news. *The good news is that there are active steps which you can take which reduce the impact of stress and which can lead to anti-depressant effects.*

## Sleep

It might seem odd to start looking at sleep as our first topic in active stress-reduction, unless of course you are one of the many cancer patients or carers suffering from insomnia. In fact insomnia is much more prevalent in cancer patients than in the general population. This is due to multiple reasons – the impact of stress and intrusive thoughts; a symptom of depression; a side effect from some cancer treatments. It may even be a physical effect caused by the cancer itself acting on the body clock via disruption of the circadian (night/day) rhythm. Insomnia can add to feelings of fatigue and exacerbate both chronic stress and depression. Tackling insomnia is, therefore, an important aspect of improving quality of life and reducing stress.

One obvious option to tackle sleep disturbances is to seek a prescription for sleeping pills – and in the past tranquilisers were often prescribed to cancer patients suffering insomnia. However, there is some evidence that patients who were prescribed tranquilisers experienced lower quality of life and in some cases these drugs worsened symptoms rather than improving them. For example one study of sleep disturbance in ovarian cancer patients found that sleep improved in the majority of patients after surgical treatment, but that those patients taking sleeping pills had a lower rate of sleep improvement compared to those not taking medication [2].

However, a number of alternatives to sleeping tablets do exist and have been shown to be effective in addressing insomnia in cancer patients and thereby improving quality of life and lowering stress levels. The two most studied interventions are based around cognitive behavioural therapy (CBT) or mindfulness-based stress reduction (MBSR) programmes which have been specifically tailored to treat insomnia. While some of these are offered as classes or group sessions at some hospitals and medical centres, there are also self-administered versions which do not require going into a hospital or medical centre to access them. Results for the self-administered courses are generally positive; for example, a small recent study found that a self-administered course of CBT for cancer patients produced improvements in all measures of sleep parameters. It also found reductions in anxiety and depressive symptoms in those who took the course, compared to a control group who did not [3]. Another trial compared patients undertaking CBT with those taking medication and found that the CBT patients reported reduced fatigue compared to the patients on medication, who showed no improvement in cancer-related fatigue [4].

A trial that compared CBT to MBSR programmes for cancer-associated insomnia, reported results in 2014, showing that both interventions produced clinically significant improvements in insomnia and stress levels. CBT was the preferred option, however, as the improvements were more rapid and longer lasting [5]. However, for patients in need of non-pharmacological solutions to insomnia either option is worth going for.

Melatonin is also an option that some cancer patients may want to consider. Melatonin is a hormone produced by the body and is essentially a regulator of our body clock – it's what signals to us that it's time for sleep. Disturbed melatonin levels may actually be a cause of sleep disturbance in some cancer patients. It is also available in tablet or liquid form and is occasionally prescribed by doctors to handle sleep problems – and in some countries it is easily available over the counter or via the internet. Strictly speaking it is not a drug, though there is a drug called ramelteon which targets the melatonin receptors and is sometimes prescribed for sleep disorders. In addition to its role in sleep, melatonin has multiple other physiological functions, including positive effects on the immune system.

A number of clinical trials have investigated the use of melatonin in cancer-related sleep disorders. A recent clinical trial in advanced breast cancer patients found that 5 mg of melatonin taken an hour before bedtime was associated with '*a significant improvement in a marker of objective sleep quality, sleep fragmentation and quantity, subjective sleep, fatigue severity, global quality of life, and social and cognitive functioning scales*' [6]. In addition it is worth noting that in another study use of melatonin in breast cancer patients was also associated with a lower risk of developing depressive symptoms [7].

Finally, many women on anti-oestrogen therapy, such as tamoxifen, suffer from severe side effects, particularly hot flushes, which can interfere significantly with sleep. In fact many end up discontinuing treatment and therefore massively increase the risks of recurrence and mortality. Some women are therefore treated either with sleeping tablets such as zopiclone, tranquilisers or anti-depressants but there is limited evidence that these provide much relief to the hot flushes and consequent sleep problems. However, hot flushes can be treated safely using low-dose progesterone tablets (megace or megestrol acetate, at a dose of 20 mg or 40 mg) [8]. The evidence for this comes from multiple clinical trials, and in fact high dose megace has also been used in the past as a cancer treatment. There have been some concerns raised in the past about an increased breast cancer risk associated with combination treatment (progesterone and oestrogen) in hormone replacement therapy (CHRT). However, there is now an increasing controversy about this although the consensus still suggests there is some degree of increased risk. Combination HRT has also been shown to *reduce* the risk of endometrial cancer [9]. What is more there is evidence that the form of progesterone is significant [10] – *there is no evidence that megace increases any breast cancer risk*. What is undeniable though is the increase in the risks associated with early discontinuation of tamoxifen treatment [11].

## Exercise

It may seem very cruel to ask stressed, fatigued or depressed cancer patients to engage in exercise, but the benefits of physical activity are so clear and so strong that it should not be discounted. The evidence exists for a wide range of cancer types, stages of disease and even from animal models investigating the biochemical effects of exercise. The message from all of these is clear – exercise helps – it reduces the impact of side effects, decreases fatigue and may even have positive effects in terms of reducing recurrence risks and improvements in long term survival.

In prostate cancer the PSA doubling time (PSADT – the length of time it takes for the level of PSA to double) is considered a standard measure of disease progression and is often used to assess whether drugs are effective in the disease or not. One very recent trial looked at the effects of exercise on PSADT, comparing one group of patients who were following a home exercise program with a matched group receiving usual care [12]. After six months of three times a week endurance training at home the PSADT had increased from 28 to 76 months, a statistically significant amount. Improvements were also noted in fasting glucose, plasma triglycerides and other physical measures. In a previous study it was noted that three hours or more per week of vigorous walking was associated with a 57% lower rate of progression than in men who walked at an easy pace for less than three hours a week [13]. A meta-analysis of trials of exercise in prostate cancer concluded:

*Current data suggest that incontinence, fitness, fatigue, body constitution, and also quality of life can be improved by clinical exercise in patients during and after prostate cancer* [14].

It is not just in prostate cancer that we see such strong results. In breast cancer too we see some very positive effects of exercise. For example, one meta-analysis looking at the role of physical activity and breast cancer outcomes concluded that:

*There is an inverse relationship between physical activity and all-cause, breast cancer-related death and breast cancer events. The current meta-analysis supports the notion that appropriate physical activity may be an important intervention for reducing death and breast cancer events among breast cancer survivors* [15].

There have also been randomised controlled studies, which have looked specifically at different forms of exercise and the impacts on levels of psychological distress, in women undergoing breast cancer chemotherapy. In one trial three groups were compared, those undergoing a standard 25 – 30 minute aerobic exercise session, those on a higher 'dose' (50 – 60 minutes per session) and those on a combined aerobic and resistance exercise session of 50 – 60 minutes, (all three times per week) [16]. The conclusion was that there was no additional benefit from doing the more intense sessions for most women and that the standard session was sufficient to reduce depressive symptoms. However, for some women with higher levels of depressive symptoms there was benefit from the higher 'dose' exercise programs.

Although I have singled out prostate and breast cancers here, there are trials reporting positive outcomes on health and stress levels in a very broad range of cancers. There is even evidence that patients with advanced cancers can benefit. For example one trial assessed the benefit of exercise in advanced lung cancer patients undergoing chemotherapy treatment [17]. Even in this patient group the trial reported improvements in physical parameters and a reduction in anxiety levels and measures of emotional well-being.

At the beginning of this chapter we talked about the hormones which are associated with stress and we can see some evidence that exercise or physical activity is associated with reductions of the levels of these hormones. An analysis of a group of breast cancer survivors looked at the levels of physical activity and the levels of cortisol and found that the women in the more active group had lower levels of circulating alpha-amylase (a marker of stress found in saliva) [18]. What is more, the high alpha-amylase/physically inactive group also had higher levels of: anger, fatigue, depression, confusion, mood disturbance and blood pressure.

The field of 'exercise oncology' is rapidly expanding and a search of currently active clinical trials reveals more than 200 trials on-going in this area. However, there is sufficient evidence available already to suggest that physical exercise leads to positive psychological outcomes. There are multiple mechanisms involved, many of them of having systemic influence. Interested readers are directed to a recent paper on this topic: 'Biological mechanisms underlying the role of physical fitness in health and resilience', which is an open access publication and freely downloadable from the Royal Society [19].

## Mindfulness Meditation

Mention has previously been made of mindfulness meditation (MM) in the section on sleep, but the topic is worth including separately as the advantages extend much beyond dealing with insomnia. Before outlining these advantages, and the evidence for them, we should perhaps spend some time explaining what MM is and, just as importantly, what it isn't.

Let's start with what MM isn't. Although the core practices involved in mindfulness are derived in large part from Buddhism, MM is not about teaching people Buddhist beliefs or any other religious belief system come to that. In fact it is not even about spirituality as such, although people with existing religious or spiritual beliefs may in fact find that it links in well with that side of their personalities – and it's as well to remember that meditation exists as a practice in Christianity, Judaism, Hinduism and Islam. However, MM works just as well in people who have no religious beliefs or who are not especially interested in spirituality.

In terms of what it is, MM can best be described as a set of simple techniques dedicated to focusing the attention internally. It is not about clearing the mind completely or about achieving a specific state of consciousness. It is the *process* of directing the attention that is important. In our increasingly stressed lives we are bombarded with stimuli, assailed by stressful situations and can find ourselves emotionally overwhelmed. Often we are anywhere but in the moment – we are thinking about the past or about the future, frequently flitting from one to the other. Mindfulness is about stepping outside of that by focusing on one specific thing in the present moment – often it is the flow of our breath while we are sitting or lying still.

MM has become increasingly recognised as a useful set of techniques in a broad range of healthcare scenarios, not just in oncology. It has also made something of a breakthrough in popular culture and there are numerous popular books, DVDs, classes and online courses dedicated to it. These are of varying quality, especially some of the do-it-yourself courses available via books and CDs. One of the better titles is 'Mindfulness: A practical guide to finding peace in a frantic world' by Professor Mark Williams and Dr Danny Penman. Available in a number of formats, the book and CD combination provides a complete mindfulness course in an accessible and effective format for those who cannot get to a class or structured course.

In a clinical setting MM is normally delivered as a structured course over a number of weeks – commonly lasting for eight weeks in the case of Mindfulness-Based Stress Reduction. A number of books, including the title recommended previously, follow a similar structure. Although common, this is not the only option, and the medical literature describes many different forms of mindfulness-based interventions, including do-it-yourself courses and much shorter courses, which condense the eight weeks down into something that lasts for one or two weeks.

There are numerous medical papers reporting results related to cancer patients and MM – for example a PubMed search on the phrase 'mindfulness cancer' currently returns more than 240 papers – and the number is rising fast. There are numerous review papers which generally report positive effects of MM on both psychological measures – particularly with regards to anxiety and depression – and on physical changes, including fatigue and biochemical markers related to immune response. In terms of psychological response there is also a recent meta-analysis, which concluded that mindfulness-based interventions were associated with statistically significant reductions in anxiety and depression in people with cancer [20].

It is worth noting that there is also some evidence that psychological interventions can have long-term positive effects on cancer-related outcomes. The best example comes from a trial that studied a cognitive-behavioural stress management intervention delivered to post-operative non-metastatic breast cancer patients. An analysis eleven years after the event showed that the women who had received this intervention had a significantly reduced risk of all-cause mortality compared to the women in the non-treatment group [21]. That means women who went on the stress management course had a much lower risk of dying from any cause (HR = 0.21; 95 % CI [0.05, 0.93]; P = 0.04). A sub-group analysis, which looked only at those women with invasive breast cancer, showed statistically significant reductions in cancer-related mortality and increased disease-free interval.

In many respects, MM is an ideal stress-reduction methodology in that it has very positive effects without the need for medication. However, it does require a willingness to engage in the process and the discipline to follow and maintain the practices that are a core part of the mindfulness approach.

## Other Strategies

In this chapter we have touched on just a few interventions which have shown some evidence of benefit in terms of stress reduction, as well as measurable improvements in symptoms, outcomes or biomarkers in the blood. But there are plenty of other interventions which are available to cancer patients and carers alike. Common examples include massage therapy, art therapy, yoga, aromatherapy and others. In many respects it does not matter what the intervention is if it works for the patient – indeed there are interventions which have very little data to support them but which may provide benefits to individual patients if they deliver reductions in feelings of distress, anxiety, loneliness and depression.

This chapter has focused on active anti-stress measures rather than on pharmacological interventions, aside from the possible use of melatonin to tackle insomnia. There are of course many drugs available which can tackle some of the psychological issues associated with cancer. These include sleeping tablets, drugs that reduce anxiety and anti-depressants. There is nothing wrong with using these, but in some respects there is an additional benefit to exercise, mindfulness and other such interventions in that they give back some feeling of control. Rather than continuing to be a passive receiver of medication, it transforms the individual to an active agent taking back some measure of control. It is even possible that this partly explains some of the positive psychological and emotional outcomes associated with these interventions.

That said there is one class of drugs, called beta-blockers, which is of increasing interest in oncology because it directly targets some of the chemical pathways associated with stress. Propranolol is the best example and the one currently with the highest level of evidence related to cancer. While propranolol is mainly used to treat high blood pressure, it is also sometimes used in the treatment of generalised anxiety disorders. What makes this drug interesting is that it tackles directly some of the main chemical pathways involved in the stress response and, as a consequence, there is some evidence that this can have a positive impact in cancer patients.

The evidence for a positive effect comes from multiple sources. Firstly there is epidemiological data that shows that there is a lower incidence of different cancers in patients being treated with propranolol for hypertension (high blood pressure). A newly published study concludes that:

*This study supports the proposition that propranolol can reduce the risk of head and neck, oesophagus, stomach, colon, and prostate cancers* [22].

In addition there have been a number of retrospective studies which have assessed the impact of propranolol in cancer treatment, with many of them finding improved outcomes. For example one 2011 study in breast cancer concluded that:

*The results provide evidence in humans to support preclinical observations suggesting that inhibiting the beta2-adrenergic signalling pathway can reduce breast cancer progression and mortality* [23].

In addition to these effects on cancer, there is also some evidence that there can be psychological benefits too. A study in 2013 compared levels of psychological stress in cancer patients also taking propranolol and those not, and found that those on propranolol had lower rates of cancer-related intrusive thoughts than similar patients not on the drug [23].

While there have been positive results in a small number of randomised clinical trials which have added propranolol to standard of care cancer treatments more evidence is required before we can expect it to become more widely used. However, studies are on-going and provide useful data which you can take to your clinicians should you wish to add this to your own cancer treatment.

## Conclusion

Stress is a natural process, but when it becomes a chronic condition it can have adverse consequences, particularly in the case of cancer. Tackling stress therefore can have important benefits, not just in the short term but in the longer term too. This chapter has outlined a number of positive steps that can be taken to reduce stress – some of them can be carried out at home, such as exercise or meditation, but many of them can also be taken in group courses or via support organisations such as Star Throwers. Social isolation is a contributor to stress, so where possible it is suggested that group activities or activities outside of the home should be taken up when they are offered.

## Summary

- Stress is a physiological and psychological reaction to immediate danger – it's part of the 'fight or flight' syndrome
- While 'natural' stress is an acute response that resolves itself once the situation that causes it has passed, it can turn into 'chronic stress' which does not resolve and may be associated with worse cancer outcomes
- There are many mechanisms for reducing psychological stress, and there is some evidence that these can have lasting and positive effects on health
- Insomnia is a common response to stress and may be exacerbated by cancer treatments. Effective mechanisms for improving sleep include CBT and mindfulness meditation. The natural hormone melatonin may also be beneficial
- Exercise has many positive effects on health, including reducing stress. There is some evidence that it has positive effects on response to cancer treatments
- Mindfulness meditation is a stress reduction technique that is easy to learn and apply
- Loneliness adds to stress, so if it is an issue look at organisations such as Star Throwers, Macmillan and others to seek help and advice

## References

1    Chida Y, Hamer M, Wardle J and Steptoe A (2008) **Do stress-related psychosocial factors contribute to cancer incidence and survival?** *Nature clinical practice. Oncology*, **5**(8), pp. 466–75.

2    Clevenger L, Schrepf A, DeGeest K, Bender D, et al. (2013) **Sleep disturbance, distress, and quality of life in ovarian cancer patients during the first year after diagnosis.** *Cancer*, **119**(17), pp. 3234–3241.

3    Casault L, Savard J, Ivers H and Savard M-H (2015) **A randomized-controlled trial of an early minimal cognitive-behavioural therapy for insomnia comorbid with cancer.** *Behaviour research and therapy*, **67**, pp. 45–54.

4    Heckler CE, Garland SN, Peoples AR, Perlis ML, et al. (2016) **Cognitive behavioral therapy for insomnia, but not armodafinil, improves fatigue in cancer survivors with insomnia: a randomized placebo-controlled trial.** *Supportive care in cancer : official journal of the Multinational Association of Supportive Care in Cancer*, **24**(5), pp. 2059–

66.

5      Garland SN, Carlson LE, Stephens AJ, Antle MC, et al. (2014) **Mindfulness-based stress reduction compared with cognitive behavioral therapy for the treatment of insomnia comorbid with cancer: a randomized, partially blinded, noninferiority trial.** *Journal of clinical oncology : official journal of the American Society of Clinical Oncology*, **32**(5), pp. 449–57.

6      Innominato PF, Lim AS, Palesh O, Clemons M, et al. (2016) **The effect of melatonin on sleep and quality of life in patients with advanced breast cancer.** *Supportive care in cancer : official journal of the Multinational Association of Supportive Care in Cancer*, **24**(3), pp. 1097–105.

7      Hansen M V., Andersen LT, Madsen MT, Hageman I, et al. (2014) **Effect of melatonin on depressive symptoms and anxiety in patients undergoing breast cancer surgery: A randomized, double-blind, placebo-controlled trial**. *Breast Cancer Research and Treatment*, **145**(3), pp. 683–695.

8      Goodwin JW, Green SJ, Moinpour CM,

Bearden JD, et al. (2008) **Phase III randomized placebo-controlled trial of two doses of megestrol acetate as treatment for menopausal symptoms in women with breast cancer: Southwest Oncology Group Study 9626.** *Journal of clinical oncology: official journal of the American Society of Clinical Oncology*, **26**(10), pp. 1650–6.

9    Chlebowski RT, Anderson GL, Sarto GE, Haque R, et al. (2016) **Continuous Combined Estrogen Plus Progestin and Endometrial Cancer: The Women's Health Initiative Randomized Trial.** *Journal of the National Cancer Institute*, **108**(3).

10    Gompel A and Plu-Bureau G (2015) **Progesterone and Synthetic Progestin Controversies.** *JAMA oncology*, **1**(7), p. 987.

11    Nichols HB, DeRoo LA, Scharf DR and Sandler DP (2015) **Risk-benefit profiles of women using tamoxifen for chemoprevention.** *Journal of the National Cancer Institute*, **107**(1), p. 354.

12    Hvid T, Lindegaard B, Winding K, Iversen P, et al. (2015) **Effect of a 2-year home-based endurance training intervention on physiological function and PSA doubling**

time in prostate cancer patients. *Cancer causes & control : CCC*.

13    Richman EL, Kenfield SA, Stampfer MJ, Paciorek A, et al. (2011) **Physical activity after diagnosis and risk of prostate cancer progression: data from the cancer of the prostate strategic urologic research endeavor.** *Cancer research*, **71**(11), pp. 3889–95.

14    Baumann FT, Zopf EM and Bloch W (2012) **Clinical exercise interventions in prostate cancer patients-a systematic review of randomized controlled trials**. *Supportive Care in Cancer*, **20**(2), pp. 221–233.

15    Lahart IM, Metsios GS, Nevill AM and Carmichael AR (2015) **Physical activity, risk of death and recurrence in breast cancer survivors: A systematic review and meta-analysis of epidemiological studies**. *Acta Oncologica*, (September 2014), pp. 1–20.

16    Courneya KS, McKenzie DC, Gelmon K, Mackey JR, et al. (2014) **A multicenter randomized trial of the effects of exercise dose and type on psychosocial distress in breast cancer patients undergoing chemotherapy.** *Cancer epidemiology,*

*biomarkers & prevention: a publication of the American Association for Cancer Research, cosponsored by the American Society of Preventive Oncology,* **23**(13), pp. 857–64.

17    Quist M, Adamsen L, Rørth M, Laursen JH, et al. (2015) **The Impact of a Multidimensional Exercise Intervention on Physical and Functional Capacity, Anxiety, and Depression in Patients With Advanced-Stage Lung Cancer Undergoing Chemotherapy.** *Integrative cancer therapies,* **14**(4), pp. 341–9.

18    Ariza-García a, Galiano-Castillo N, Cantarero-Villanueva I, Fernández-Lao C, et al. (2013) **Influence of physical inactivity in psychophysiological state of breast cancer survivors.** *European journal of cancer care,* **22**(6), pp. 738–45.

19    Silverman MN and Deuster PA (2014) **Biological mechanisms underlying the role of physical fitness in health and resilience.** *Interface focus,* **4**(5), p. 20140040.

20    Zhang M-F, Wen Y-S, Liu W-Y, Peng L-F, et al. (2015) **Effectiveness of Mindfulness-based Therapy for Reducing Anxiety and**

**Depression in Patients With Cancer: A Meta-analysis.** *Medicine*, **94**(45), pp. e0897–0.

21  Stagl JM, Lechner SC, Carver CS, Bouchard LC, et al. (2015) **A randomized controlled trial of cognitive-behavioral stress management in breast cancer: survival and recurrence at 11-year follow-up.** *Breast cancer research and treatment.*

22  Chang P-Y, Huang W-Y, Lin C-L, Huang T-C, et al. (2015) **Propranolol Reduces Cancer Risk: A Population-Based Cohort Study.** *Medicine*, **94**(27), p. e1097.

23  Barron TI, Connolly RM, Sharp L, Bennett K and Visvanathan K (2011) **Beta blockers and breast cancer mortality: a population-based study.** *Journal of clinical oncology : official journal of the American Society of Clinical Oncology*, **29**(19), pp. 2635–44.

# Cancer and Diet

## Introduction

The topic of cancer and diet is one of the most difficult and contested areas in oncology, but it's also one that is of enormous interest to patients, doctors and researchers alike. It's not difficult to understand this level of interest. On the one hand there is an enormous amount of research looking at the role that diet plays in cancer initiation - are there diets which are better or worse when it comes to developing cancer? And on the other hand, and perhaps of more interest to readers of this book, there is the question of whether certain foods help fight cancer once it has developed, or which can be beneficial during treatment. Are diets which stop cancer forming in the first place also good for stopping it once it has started? These are tricky questions which will we try and address later in this chapter.

Before we start looking at this in detail, however, let's just step back and consider what we know about diet in general. Even a cursory glance at the media shows a huge level of disagreement and uncertainty about pretty much every facet of the relationship between diet and health. There are numerous competing diets all claiming to be based on sound science: the Atkins, modified Atkins, 5:2, paleo and more. Each is backed up with a scientific rationale and promoted using books, videos and websites. We see also that certain foods win popular acclaim as 'super-foods' only for them to be dismissed later as being unhealthy or not all they are cracked up to be.

It is not just the mass media and companies selling diets or dietary products that are to blame. Very often stories about diets and health originate in scientific research and the results of clinical trials. In fact it is increasingly apparent that even some of the cornerstones of official dietary advice from governments are open to serious dispute. For example, for many years the official advice has been to reduce saturated fats from the diet because of the link to 'unhealthy' cholesterol levels and the risk of heart attacks. Yet even this, which has been considered fundamental to official dietary advice for decades, is now increasingly being challenged and not supported by all of the evidence [1–3].

With that in mind, it should be no surprise that there are huge uncertainties when it comes to diet and cancer. However, even in the face of this state of affairs there are certain things that we can say, particularly when it comes to addressing a number of common misconceptions about food and cancer. In addressing each of these issues in turn we can explore some of the underlying biology of cancer and diet and look at the evidence where it exists. Although this process necessarily involves debunking some popular misconceptions it is not meant to be an exercise in negativity. It is certainly not the intention to say that diet is unimportant and that it doesn't matter what you eat and drink. In fact the opposite is the case – for many people with cancer, both those undergoing treatment and those in remission, taking control of diet has a hugely empowering effect. These positive effects are important, both physically and psychologically, and are therefore to be encouraged.

## Organic vs non-organic

On the face of it the case for eating organic foods should be very straightforward, particularly for cancer patients. However, on closer examination the case in favour is not so clear. Firstly it is a commonly believed that organic produce is grown without the use of *any* herbicides or insecticides – this is not actually the case. Organic food uses certain 'approved' pesticides, including rotenone and pyrethrin, some of which are considered carcinogenic (cancer-causing) or otherwise hazardous to health. More worrying still, for those cancer patients who are selecting organic foods to avoid pesticide residues, is a report of a study by the United States Department of Agriculture in 2012 that found that 4% of organic food samples had pesticide residues above the 5% EPA limit. Technically meant they would have failed the organic certification they carried [4]. And it is not just in fruit and vegetables that there are few differences; in the case of meat, a study published in April 2015 showed that there were minimal differences between organic and non-organic chicken, lamb and beef in terms of residues, concluding that:

*'Strikingly, the consumption of organically produced meat does not diminish this carcinogenic risk, but on the contrary, it seems to be even higher, especially that associated with lamb consumption.'* [5]

In addition to concern about pesticides and other toxic chemicals, there is also a widespread belief that organic vegetables contain higher levels of nutrients than non-organic. Again, however, there is very little published scientific evidence to support this assertion. For example a systematic review published in the Annals of Internal Medicine in 2012 found that:

'*The published literature lacks strong evidence that organic foods are significantly more nutritious than conventional foods.*' [6]

What about organic diets and the risk of developing cancer? A study published in the British Journal of Cancer, by Dr Kathryn Bradbury and co-workers as part of the Million Women Study, (funded by Cancer Research UK and the Medical Research Council), tracked 623,080 middle-aged British women for almost ten years. It looked at their pattern of organic food consumption and the incidence of sixteen different cancer types, as well as overall cancer incidence [7]. Based on their reported eating habits the women were put into three groups: never, sometimes, or usually/always eating organic food. The headline result showed that eating organic was not associated with overall cancer incidence one way or another (in fact there was a tiny increased overall risk of about 3%, but it's the sort of weak or 'noisy' result due to random effects that one can ignore). Look at the specific cancer types and the results are mixed, with some showing increased or decreased risks, but again nothing to be alarmed (or pleased) about. Notably the numbers show that there is an apparent 21% decrease in non-Hodgkins lymphoma risk among the women who reported usually or always eating organic food. But this has to be balanced against an apparent 9% increase in the risk of breast cancer and a 37% increase in the risk of developing a soft tissue sarcoma. Of course, these are relative risks; the risk of developing a soft tissue sarcoma is very small (except for people with a genetic cancer condition called Li Fraumeni Syndrome), so a 37% increase on a very small risk still leaves a very small risk.

Indirect evidence can also come from looking at the health risks associated with working with the chemicals in food that we are most concerned about. A recently published paper looked at the incidence of cancer in agricultural workers in France during the period 2005 – 2009 (the AGRICAN study). It reported that overall agricultural workers were healthier than the general population, with reduced cancer incidence compared to the general population in the same areas [8]. However, a later study suggested an increased prostate cancer risk in some areas and some farming activities [9].

What this means is that there is little solid evidence for health benefits coming from eating organic foods. Given the additional costs involved, it may be more beneficial to spend the extra to increase the intake of vegetables and fresh foods and cut down on processed foods and ready meals instead. What is more, it is also advisable that all fresh fruit and vegetables be thoroughly washed before use – and this applies as much to organic produce as non-organic. In fact organic fruit and vegetables may be at increased risk of microbial contamination because they are fertilised with animal manures which contain high levels of faecal bacteria and animal hormones.

For those who are interested in organic diets one very positive step is 'growing your own'. Not only does this mean you have some control in the growing conditions, including the use of pesticides and herbicides, it means you benefit from food that is freshly harvested, with all the pleasure that comes from eating the fruits of your own labours. There are positive effects physically from the effort involved in gardening, but also the psychological benefits that come from gardening. Believe it or not there have even been studies in cancer patients and survivors, which have shown positive evidence of benefit in health and well-being from gardening [10]. And for those without access to a garden, there are plenty of community garden schemes and allotments, which also have the benefit of social interactions and positive psychological effects from being able to 'switch off ' from cancer and engage the attention on something totally different.

## The cancer-glucose connection

A key component of many 'anticancer diets' is the advice to reduce sugar intake - in fact this is probably just about the only thing that diets as diverse as the Gerson, Budwig, paleo, macrobiotics, Atkins and 5:2 have in common. The reason is simple and often grounded in an understanding of an important aspect of tumour cell metabolism called the 'Warburg Effect'.

All cells, not just cancer cells, need nutrients to survive and there are different 'fuels' which cells can use as sources for the generation of ATP – which is the 'energy' molecule used to drive chemical reactions in the cell. There are two main metabolic pathways which cells can use:

- oxidative phosphorylation – this is the more efficient pathway used in most cells in the body
- glycolysis – which breaks down glucose to generate the ATP the cell needs.

Normally our cells use oxidative phosphorylation, (also called *aerobic respiration* because it depends on oxygen), however, there are times when cells can switch to glycolysis, (also called *anaerobic respiration* because it doesn't depend on oxygen). For example at rest our muscle cells use oxidative phosphorylation to generate the energy they need.

78

But, when they suddenly have to spring into action they can switch to glycolysis. In other words the cells can become glycolytic when they undergo intense and sustained exercise and the supply of blood and oxygen can't meet the demand for energy – in running for example. A side effect of glycolysis is the production of lactate, which you can feel when it builds up in your muscles after a hard run, for example. When the exercise is over, and you return to a resting state, the muscle cells revert back to using oxidative phosphorylation again.

German scientist Otto Warburg, who won the Nobel Prize in Medicine in 1931, discovered that cancer cells, which have higher energy demands than non-cancer cells, use the glycolytic pathway to drive their increased growth rates and energy needs. They do this even in the presence of adequate oxygen. In fact the 'Warburg hypothesis' is that this metabolic switch to glycolysis is one of the main causes of cancer rather than being a *consequence* of the disease. In any case glycolysis provides a number of advantages to tumour cells, including the ability to survive and prosper in low-oxygen conditions. It contributes to an acidic microenvironment that is toxic to non-cancer cells and it provides many intermediate by-products that enable cells to rapidly divide.

One result of the Warburg effect is an increased need for glucose by tumours. There is evidence from test tube, animal and human studies that reducing the level of glucose in the blood may slow tumour growth and in some cases even cause cancer cells to die. It is also commonly observed in some cancers that patients experience an increase in high blood glucose (hyper-glycemia) as a *consequence* of their disease. There is also some evidence that high blood glucose is associated with poorer outcomes in cancer. Therefore there is a huge level of interest in drugs which can impact the level of blood glucose or interfere with the Warburg effect, including the anti-diabetic drug metformin and the experimental drugs dichloroacetate (DCA) and 2-Deoxy-D-glucose. There is also much research interest in trying to assess the role of dietary change in cancer too, mostly with respect to changes in blood glucose levels.

In terms of diet, therefore, is there anything we can do? Obviously one simple change is to try and reduce the level of glucose in the blood by changing the diet. To do this means not just cutting down on sugar – though that is an obvious start – but it also means cutting back on those foods which the body breaks down into glucose. That means cutting back on carbohydrates, including high-carb foods such as pasta, rice, bread, potatoes, sweets, sugary drinks, fruit juices and more. It is interesting that many diets which are promoted as anticancer diets for different reasons actually lead to a reduction of carbohydrate intake. The most extreme versions of this include the ketogenic diet, which eliminates practically all carbohydrates. Other, less extreme diets, such as the Atkins, Budwig or 5:2 diets also include significant levels of carbohydrate reduction.

The clinical evidence on carbohydrate reduction, or caloric reduction in general, is still limited but on the positive side. For example there is some evidence that the ketogenic diet has positive effects in glioblastoma in conjunction with standard treatments [11]. There are a number of clinical trials investigating this at the moment, in other cancers as well as in brain tumours. It should be noted that the ketogenic diet is extremely hard to stick to, so there is intense activity researching other diets that have similar effects on blood glucose but which are easier to adhere to.

However, we should sound a note of caution that in recent years our understanding of cancer cell metabolism has expanded. It is now known that not all cancers exhibit the Warburg effect. Some cancers are able to metabolise glutamine, acetate, fats and other alternative molecules. Professor Michael

Lisanti and his colleagues have also described a 'reverse Warburg effect', in which cancer cells *induce* glycolysis in surrounding non-cancer cells, and then use the by-products of this to fuel themselves [12]. In patient samples, from a range of different cancer types, they have described tumours with different metabolic 'compartments' in which distinct populations of cells exist in *complex metabolic relationships* which go well beyond a simplistic view of the Warburg effect. It is increasingly accepted that cancers display 'metabolic plasticity', in which different populations of cancer cells in tumours adapt and change their metabolism in response to the changing availability of different nutrients and oxygen.

The upshot of this more nuanced view of cancer metabolism is that it is unlikely that dietary interventions *alone* can defeat established or metastatic disease. However, the current weight of evidence does suggest that *dietary change may be beneficial*, particularly in the case of hyper-glycemia, obesity, metabolic syndrome and so on. Looking at the range of clinical trials in this area, the major focus does appear to be on low-carbohydrate diets, including ketogenic, modified Atkins, 5:2 and others.

## Fasting

One dietary approach that has gained increasing levels of both public and scientific interest is fasting – sometimes also known as caloric restriction in the more technical discussions. In the past some people have been attracted to the idea of intermittent fasting as a way of 'detoxifying' the body. The idea is that cancers are driven by an accumulation of environmental toxins in the body and that fasting is a way for the body to clear these out. Detox diets, many of which include periods of fasting, have become popular not just for cancer patients but also for many other chronic medical conditions. However, there is little scientific support for the theory, not even for the fundamental premise that there are toxins which are stored in our tissues and contribute to ill-health. In fact 'toxins' is rather a vague term in this context and it includes food additives, household cleaning materials, pollutants in the air and environment, even the by-products of our normal metabolism. In many cases the whole 'detox' idea has become a marketing strategy to sell different products, from herbal teas to books to spa days and vitamin and mineral supplements. There is a good article, in plain non-technical language, which describes the lack of evidence for detox here: https://www.sciencebasedmedicine.org/the-detox-scam-how-to-spot-it-and-how-to-avoid-it/.

However, one of the main drivers of the increasing scientific interest in fasting is nothing to do with vague notions of 'detox' and everything to do with an increased understanding of metabolic processes in the body, particularly with regards to tumour metabolism. Yes, we're back to the Warburg Effect and the impact of glucose on tumour growth. As with the ketogenic diet, intermittent fasting is about cutting down massively on the supply of nutrients to tumours. What is surprising though is that the effect of fasting appears to be due to much more than simply cutting down on carbohydrates.

One effect that has been described in the scientific literature is called 'differential stress resistance'. A team of scientists, led by Dr Valter Longo, has been most active in this area. These researchers have shown in test tube and mice experiments that fasting, which they term 'short term starvation', protected normal cells from the effects of chemotherapy [13]. They treated mice that had neuroblastoma tumours with the chemotherapy drug etoposide, with one group experiencing fasting conditions during treatment and another having a normal diet. All were compared to untreated mice as a control group. The results showed that fasting reduced the number of mice who died due to treatment toxicity, and increased the survival time. The explanation was that the fasting – which lasted for 48 hours – protected the normal cells from the stress of chemotherapy while it increased the effect of chemo on the cancer cells. The same team carried out a range of other experiments using different chemo drugs and different cancer types and found similar results. Later work showed that in addition to exploiting the better stress resistance of normal cells, fasting also had very positive effects on the immune system [14].

As always we have to be cautious in interpreting results from animal models to humans. But there is some evidence that the differential stress resistance effect does occur in people too. A case series report was published on ten patients undergoing chemotherapy for a range of different cancers who fasted before and immediately after treatment [15]. The results showed that fasting led to lower levels of side effects, lower tiredness and, where the data was available, it showed no signs of interfering with the effectiveness of the treatment. A case series report is not a randomised clinical trial (please see the chapter on assessing clinical evidence for more details of the difference between the two), so we have to wait for the results of the clinical trials currently taking place before we can draw firm conclusions as to the value of fasting. One very small trial in breast cancer patients, in the Netherlands, has confirmed the positive effects in terms of chemo impact on bone marrow and other blood markers [16]. To date no clinical trial has reported results in terms of actual survival or disease outcomes.

While clinical trials are on-going, there is also much research to see if the positive effects of fasting can be had without incurring the negative effects. These include the symptoms of fasting, such as dizziness, headache and tiredness, and the effects on body weight. The latter is of particular concern because loss of body weight is also associated with a serious condition called cancer cachexia. This potentially deadly condition is often associated with advanced cancer, and so there is a fear among some doctors that fasting may help bring this on or make it worse when it exists.

One response to this is to look at special diets which mirror the effects of fasting. These are termed 'fasting mimetic diets' or 'fast mimicking diets' and there are a number currently in development and being tested in randomised controlled trials. The trick is to discover what combination of foods/nutrients can replicate the positive effects of fasting but also make it easier to cope with the effects of hunger. Fasting, we have to remember, cuts out not just the carbohydrates that ketogenic diets target, but also proteins, fats, amino acids and so on.

So far we have only talked about fasting in terms of cancer patients undergoing chemotherapy treatment. Is there anything for those people in remission or in high risk groups? Again we have to look at animal experiments first, as this is where most of the research has been. The evidence here is very strong and it shows that even in mice with a genetic predisposition to cancer, similar to people with Li Fraumeni Syndrome or BRCA1/BRCA2 carriers, intermittent fasting has been shown to reduce the cancer incidence rate [17]. However, the effect has yet to be shown in humans, although there are some trials planned in which fasting and exercise are combined to see if it can have an impact on cancer incidence in women at high risk of the disease.

While this is a very active and interesting area of research, with significant potential to make a meaningful difference to cancer outcomes, the data so far is only suggestive and not at all definitive. However, for those who are interested in exploring this option in their own treatment, there are a number of things to keep in mind. The first is that the research shows that the effects are related to intermittent fasting, not prolonged fasts. Most of the work has used fasts of 48 – 60 hours. For chemo patients the timing should be that the fast begins at least 24 hours before administration of the chemo, and continues afterwards. Secondly it's important to remain well hydrated – the clinical trial protocols, for example, allow water, coffee and tea (without sugar or milk). It's also important to keep track of weight change. While fasting will lower your weight, it should come back up again afterwards – a sustained and continued loss of weight is not something you should be aiming for unless you have a serious weight problem (see section on weight later in this chapter).

## Acid and alkaline foods

One of the side effects of high rates of glycolysis is the production of lactate and lactic acid, leading, in the case of cancer, to the build-up of an acidic tissue environment around solid tumours. This acidic environment provides a number of survival advantages to tumours:

- it degrades non-cancer tissues
- it stops chemotherapy drugs getting to cancer cells
- it helps subvert the immune system and so on.

What is more interesting is that in test tubes and in animal experiments it has been shown that reducing this acidic microenvironment slows tumour growth and in some cases leads to tumour shrinkage.

Currently there are a number of clinical trials which are looking at the use of drugs to target these tumour-associated acidic areas. In some cases the drugs being investigated are repurposed antacids (see the chapter on drug repurposing for details on what this is), including common drugs such as omeprazole, lansoprazole and other proton pump inhibitors (PPIs). Other work has looked at the use of sodium bicarbonate solution, alone and in combination with other drugs. To date the results have been interesting but inconclusive. However, should these results prove positive then we will have another weapon in the anticancer armoury, and one associated with low cost and low levels of toxicity.

Can we do something with diet to change the levels of acidity around tumours? There is certainly a lot of interest in this from patients, and indeed not just cancer patients. Judging by the numerous websites and books promoting 'alkalizing' diets and supplements, this is of interest to lots of people concerned about a wide range of health issues. The rationale is simple enough – our cells and tissues are adapted to an alkaline environment; aside from the extremely acidic conditions in the digestive system, areas of acidosis tend to be associated with cancer, kidney damage, infection and so on. Even in the stomach, excess acid is associated with ulcers, reflux and so on.

Therefore there is no shortage of advice on which foods are considered acid-forming and those which are considered alkaline-forming. There are in fact numerous diets which aim to correct a perceived acid-alkaline imbalance through particular food regimens – common approaches include food combining, avoiding certain 'acid-forming' foods, eating 'alkali forming' foods, juicing and more. Many of these diets offer conflicting advice and in fact the same foods may be described as acid-forming or alkali-forming by different websites.

How can you tell whether your diet is having an effect in changing your acid-alkaline balance? As you may remember from your school science classes, acidity/alkalinity is measured on the pH scale, with a value between 6.6 – 7.3 classed as neutral, lower values more acid and higher values more alkaline (also called more 'basic'). Blood has a pH value of 7.4, battery acid has pH values below 1.0, and bleach is strongly alkaline with a pH above 12.0. As you can see, extreme acids and alkalis are dangerous, toxic substances. The simple way of measuring pH is to use litmus paper which changes colour when put into contact with acid or alkaline solutions – the paper turns red with acid, blue with alkaline. So, it would seem that there's a simple test for checking your balance – just buy some litmus paper strips and off you go. Unfortunately it's not that simple…

The simplest way of using litmus paper is to test your urine – it's easy enough to pee on a strip of litmus paper and then read off the pH value from a colour chart. However, this simply tells you what the pH is of your urine, which is not the same as the pH value of your blood. The problem is that the pH value of your urine can spike up or down very quickly and in response to changes in diet but this change does not reflect what is going on in the major tissues of the body. However, the body has evolved all sorts of control and feedback systems to maintain the pH at around 7.4 for the blood and tissues. There is very little evidence that changing the pH of your urine has any effect on the pH of your whole body.

However, many of the acid-alkaline diets restrict the intake of sugary drinks, processed foods, meat and so on, and increase the intake of selected fruit and vegetables. In this way they may have quite positive effects independent of any changes on systemic pH.

Finally, it should be understood that it is the *tumours themselves which create an acidic environment* as a by-product of their metabolism. It is not the acid that forms the tumours. Furthermore, the most viable clinical research investigating the modification of the acid environment around tumours uses targeted drugs or systemic buffers (a chemical which neutralises acid or alkali changes, such as sodium bicarbonate solution) to do this, *not* dietary change.


## Cancer and dairy products

Another incredibly contentious topic is the role of dairy produce: in cancer initiation, during treatment and in the risk of disease recurrence. This is particularly the case with cancers that have a strong hormonal component: breast, endometrial, ovarian and prostate. Feelings on this issue run very high, with some convinced that the merest hint of dairy produce is bad, and others equally convinced that there is no danger from milk and milk products at all.

If we look at the data then the picture is decidedly complex. Let's look at the risk of cancer initiation first – is there a danger signal that we can pick up from looking at data from lots of past and present cancer patients (this approach is called epidemiology)? Numerous studies and meta-analyses show conflicting evidence. Even when we look at a single cancer type there are studies which come to opposing conclusions, sometimes based on the same kind of raw data. Part of the problem is that we're using a label such as 'breast cancer' or 'ovarian cancer' as if it is a distinct and homogeneous entity – but the fact is that each of these is a group of different diseases, often with multiple subtypes, each with distinct behaviours and drivers. We are doing the same when we talk about 'dairy products' – again there are numerous types of product, including high/low fat milk, hard and soft cheeses, butter, different types of cream, fermented products such as yoghurt and so on. Each has a different chemical make-up, with different levels of fats, calcium, proteins and other nutrients. Finally, there is evidence that the effects of dairy intake vary both by gender, culture and the age of intake – for example milk intake may have a different impact on teenage girls versus post-menopausal women.

The upshot of this complex picture is that it's hard to be categorical about the health impacts of dairy produce on cancer. Some studies show protective effects in certain cancers and slightly increased risks in others. Yoghurt generally has positive associations with reduced cancer incidence or outcomes whereas high fat cheese sometimes has positive and sometimes negative effects.

Should cancer patients avoid dairy? There is not enough evidence to say 'yes' or 'no' with any real level of confidence. However, a prudent approach would be to look at dairy intake in the context of the total diet and lifestyle. A high-fat, high-dairy, high-carb and low exercise life-style is likely to be associated with poor health independently of cancer – and in fact obesity is one of the biggest modifiable risk factors associated with cancer incidence and progression. And, it's worth pointing out that switching some of that dairy intake to yoghurt might be high on the list of things to consider.

## Is meat good or bad?

As with dairy, so with meat intake – this is an incredibly complex area with conflicting data and advice. First we have to look at the difference between cancer *initiation* and *progression* – we cannot assume that these have the same drivers. Secondly we have the issues of what we mean by meat – one commonly used distinction is between red meat and non-red meat – these are often assessed separately in epidemiological studies. There is also a distinction made between processed and non-processed meat, but even these distinctions vary across studies. For example many studies include sausages in the processed meats category, but in the UK sausages are not typically made using cured or processed meats. Further complicating matters is the method of cooking meat, which also has an influence on the biological effects it has. And again we have the same problem when talking about cancer in general or even breast cancer specifically – there are many types and subtypes of the disease, with different drivers and biological behaviour.

In spite of these complexities there has been much media attention paid to recent announcements that meat or processed meats are potentially carcinogenic. In some cases misleading media stories have compared the cancer risks of meat consumption to those of smoking – this is actually very far from the truth and those media outlets that have carried the story in those terms have done the public a huge disservice.

It may be instructive to tease out the data of this particular example in some detail as it illustrates some important points. The source of the story comes from a press release issued by International Agency for Research on Cancer (https://www.iarc.fr/en/media-centre/pr/2015/pdfs/pr240_E.pdf), which is an agency of the World Health Organisation. This was issued in connection with a full meta-analysis that concluded that red meat was *'probably carcinogenic'* based on limited evidence in colorectal cancer, and that processed meat was carcinogenic based on *'sufficient evidence in humans that the consumption of processed meat causes colorectal cancer'*. The press release tried to quantify this last statement with an example: *'each 50 gram portion of processed meat eaten daily increases the risk of colorectal cancer by 18%'*. There was a huge flurry of media attention that followed, particularly with regards to the processed meats.

But looking at the data in more detail gives a slightly different perspective. Firstly the data behind these statements actually comes from a study published in 2011 which found that the risks applied to colon cancer specifically, rather than colorectal (i.e. there was no association with rectal cancer) [18]. Secondly the actual numbers reported were:

*When analyzed separately, colorectal cancer risk was related to intake of fresh red meat (RR [relative risk] (for 100 g/day increase) = 1.17, 95% CI = 1.05-1.31) and processed meat (RR (for 50 g/day increase) = 1.18, 95% CI = 1.10-1.28). Similar results were observed for colon cancer, but for rectal cancer, no significant associations were observed.*

The first thing to note is that the risks are reported as *relative risks*, (in other words as an *increase* of risk), rather than as the absolute risk itself. For example if people in one group get cancer at the rate of 1 in 100, and people in another group get cancer at a rate of 2 in 100 the relative risk is almost 100% even though the absolute risk is still only 2%. Secondly, the 95% confidence intervals, which measure the uncertainty in the results are actually quite wide, and in the case of the red meat result the lower value is very close to one (which would mean no increased risk). There is a smaller confidence interval for the processed meat results, which means that we can be more confident in that result, which suggests that the incremental risk for each additional intake of 50 g (about two slices of bacon) per day of processed meat is in the range 10% - 28%, with the most likely value being 18%, which is the example quoted in the press release and media stories.

What does this mean in practice? Well, relative risk is relative to the background risk – in other words the risk of *anyone* getting colorectal cancer. This absolute risk varies by location (even in the UK there is a regional difference between England, Scotland and Wales), age, gender, family history and so on. Ignoring this and taking the life-time risk for a man or woman in the UK of developing colorectal cancer we get a number of 61 per 1000 people in 2012 (an absolute risk of 6.1%). If this increases by 18% we get we get a figure for *life-time* risk of around 72 per 1000 people. Most people would agree that this increase of 11 per 1000 people across a life-time is not as alarming as that headline figure of 18%

suggests. It certainly does not mean that you have an 18% chance of developing colorectal cancer in your lifetime.

In fact the same analysis also compared those with the highest and lowest consumption of red meat and the risk of colorectal cancer and calculated the increased risk of higher intake. For red meat consumption the figure was 1.10 (95% CI, 1.00 – 1.21) per additional 100 g per day, and for processed meat the figures were 1.17 (95% CI, 1.09 – 1.25). Again, in the context of absolute risks these are not as alarming as the figures might suggest.

What about those who eat no meat at all? There are many people who advocate vegetarian or vegan diets in terms of positive health benefits. However, the evidence is mixed, as it often is when it comes to looking at food and health. A recent analysis looked at mortality in the UK for vegetarians and different matched groups of non-vegetarians (meat eaters, low-meat eaters and fish-eaters) [19]. The study also looked at a subgroup of vegans separately too, which meant that in some of the analyses there were five different diet groups that could be compared against each other. The headline figure showed no significant difference in overall mortality between these groups, but there were some interesting patterns when it came to cancer mortality. When the five diet groups were compared for cancer-related mortality the only group with a statistically significant lower risk were fish eaters, although there were hints that the low-meat and vegetarian groups had lower risks than the regular meat or vegan groups. In looking at analyses by types of cancer the results are more nuanced, in this set of results the study authors looked at the data for vegans and vegetarians as a single combined group. For most types of cancer there were no real differences, but for pancreatic cancer the results showed that the combined vegan and vegetarian group and the low meat groups had lower risk than the regular meat group. For lymphatic or haematological cancers the vegan and vegetarian group had the lower risk. All that we can conclude from the study is that there is no fixed pattern of health benefit to one dietary pattern across all disease groups. While there may be many good reasons for adopting a vegetarian or vegan diet, lower overall mortality is not one of them according to this data.

However, all of this is not to say that eating huge amounts of meat is necessarily a great thing to do in terms of cancer. As with the advice when it comes to dairy, the best advice might be to practice moderation.

## Alcohol

Can alcohol be good for you if you have cancer or are in remission? For many years the obvious answer was a clear NO. Many authorities list alcohol as a risk factor in cancer development, and in fact the American Institute of Cancer Research suggests that even small amounts of alcohol pose some cancer risk and therefore recommends not drinking at all. Epidemiological evidence suggests that the risks are in fact dose dependent – the more that you drink, and the longer that you drink, the higher the risk. There is also variation by cancer type: head and neck, oesophageal, liver and some types of breast cancer are most associated with alcohol as a risk factor.

This clear message has become muddied in recent years by a fairly widespread belief that red wine has potent anticancer properties. This is true enough. Red wine is rich in polyphenols: flavonoids, anthocyanins, tannins, stilbenes, procyanidins and many more. In particular there has been a huge amount of interest in resveratrol, a stilbenoid which is found in grape skins and in blueberries, raspberries and other berries. Much has also been made of the 'French paradox' – the finding that despite higher levels of saturated fat and alcohol consumption than in other advanced economies, the French seem to suffer lower rates of cardiovascular disease. This apparent paradox has been attributed by many people to the protective effects of red wine, and in some cases specifically to the effects of resveratrol.

There has subsequently been a huge amount of research focused on the anticancer properties of resveratrol. However, despite some interesting data in test tubes and to a lesser extent in mice, there is little evidence to show any measurable effect in humans. Resveratrol is a compound that has very low levels of bioavailability, simply put the body is very good at metabolising the compound so that only a tiny fraction of it passes into the circulation. Even high dose supplements do not produce the kinds of levels that are used in test tube experiments (please refer to the chapter on assessing preclinical data for a general discussion of this issue). Furthermore, it now appears that red wine actually contains very low levels of resveratrol, suggesting that if there are cardiovascular benefits associated with moderate red wine consumption it is likely down to some other factor.

When we look at human data on red wine consumption and cancer the story is often disappointing, particularly for those of us who enjoy an occasional glass of the stuff. For example a 2010 study assessed moderate red wine consumption to see if there was a protective effect on colorectal cancer incidence in men – but the data showed no association [20]. The same authors analysed the data in relation to prostate cancer and found the same lack of association [21]. However, we should note that this means there was no association the other way too. So, red wine consumption didn't provide a cancer-protective effect, but neither did it have a harmful effect.

There are also a few studies which have found a positive effect for alcohol consumption on cancer risk. For example a recent meta-analysis found that *moderate* red wine consumption was associated with a lowered risk of ovarian cancer [22]. However, the majority of findings find either no relationship or a negative one. The most positive thing that can be said is that there may be a relationship between alcohol consumption, particularly red wine, and overall mortality. At the wider population level while there may be an increased risk of dying from cancer, this is balanced by a decreased risk of dying from cardiovascular disease.

As with many diet related topics, there is no real clear picture emerging from the data. If there is one thing that nearly everyone agrees on it is that *heavy* drinking increases the risk of developing cancer in the first place, and increases the risk of recurrence and disease progression. It *really* is not a good idea.

There is also evidence that the combination of smoking and drinking is a bad one – remember smoking is the single most modifiable risk factor there is when it comes to cancer. It is also clear that red wine is not, in general, a potent anti-cancer weapon. But it is not clear either that it is especially dangerous when consumed in moderation – by which is meant around a glass of wine a day (175 ml) or less.

The bottom line is that an occasional drink, particularly of red wine, does not appear to be an especially dangerous or risky thing to do.

## Super-foods

There are numerous dietary interventions related to cancer that are based on the idea that there are 'super foods', with many people convinced that these are a key part of an 'anticancer diet'. The basis for this idea is that certain foods contain high levels of chemicals which have shown anticancer activity in laboratory experiments, including some in animal models of cancer. Examples include broccoli (sulforaphane), tomatoes (lycopene), berries (anthocyanins), garlic (allicin), green tea (EGCG), turmeric (curcumin) and so on. Indeed there are many foods with high levels of specific nutrients that do seem to display anticancer activity at sufficiently high levels in test tube experiments. However, in many cases the laboratory experiments do not use food sources but purified extracts – and there are numerous problems with extrapolating from what goes on in a test tube or petri dish and what goes on in people (see the chapter on assessing data from preclinical studies for more details). Similarly many of the animal experiments are not at all realistic – the mice or rats are often injected with purified extracts rather than taking them in the diet.

While they are few and far between, we are starting to see some interesting data coming out of clinical trials. For example, in one trial looking at the influence of diet on cardiovascular disease in women (the PREDIMED trial), there were significantly fewer instances of breast cancer in women assigned to a Mediterranean diet with extra virgin olive oil and women assigned to a Mediterranean diet with nuts, compared to those assigned to a low fat diet [23]. A trial in men with prostate cancer evaluated the effect of a supplement containing pomegranate, green tea, broccoli and turmeric (all rich in polyphenols). It found a significant short-term, favourable effect on the percentage rise in PSA (prostate specific antigen) in men managed with active surveillance and watchful waiting treated with the food supplement compared to a similarly managed control group treated with a dummy tablet (called a placebo) [24]. Another trial reported that eating nuts was associated with a lowered risk of developing cancer, particularly colorectal, endometrial and pancreatic cancers [25]. Other trials have reported positive results for omega 3 fatty acids, curcumin, walnuts, probiotics, green tea and other food-derived agents.

However, these trials are generally small, short term and report on specific markers in the bloodstream (normally referred to as biomarkers) rather than on end-points such as recurrence rate, disease-free survival or overall survival (these terms are discussed in more detail in a later chapter). While these results are hopeful indicators that there may be positive effects on longer term outcomes, they are not yet strong enough to conclude that taking supplements or eating high amounts of specific 'super foods' are an effective anticancer strategy by *themselves*. We also have to balance this with numerous clinical trials which have failed to find *any* positive effects from some of the same foods and nutrients.

So, while the idea that some foods have specific anticancer properties is appealing, there is as yet insufficient evidence to say that any of them have a strong enough effect in isolation. A 'super food' is more of a marketing term than anything else. That said, anyone interested in looking at a range of foods which have some laboratory evidence in their favour should look at the book 'Foods To Fight Cancer' by the research scientists Richard Beliveau and Denis Gingras. This is a very accessible, readable book on the whole issue of food and cancer.

## Weight

While there is much dispute about most of the topics we've looked at so far, there is one area where there is a strong argument for making a change – and that is when it comes to extremes of body weight. By extremes we mean not just extremely high weights – obesity in other words – but also for those who are extremely underweight. Both extremes are associated with worse medical outcomes, and in the case of obesity it is also associated with an increased risk of some types of cancer developing in the first place.

Before looking at the details we need to digress first and talk a little bit about definitions. Obesity is most often defined in terms of the body-mass index (BMI). This is calculated by dividing the body mass (weight in kg) by the square of the height (the height, measured in metres, multiplied by itself). For example, an adult with a height of 1.75 metres (5' 9'') and weight of 70 kg (around 11 stone or just over 154 lbs):

$$BMI = 70 / (1.75 \times 1.75) = 70 / 3.06 = 22.9$$

The World Health Organisation publishes a set of internationally recognised categories of weight organised by BMI. The main categories are:

| Classification | BMI (kg/m$^2$) |
|---|---|
| Underweight | <18.50 |
| Normal range | 18.50 - 24.99 |
| Overweight | ≥25.00 |
| Obese | ≥30.00 |
| Obese class I | 30.00 - 34.99 |
| Obese class II | 35.00 - 39.99 |
| Obese class III | ≥40.00 |

While these categories are used in most areas of medicine, there are a number of rather obvious problems with BMI as a measure. The first and most obvious is that BMI tells us very little about body composition. Two people may differ completely in their physical make-up and yet have exactly the same BMI – for example one person may have lots of excess fat and another person may have a lot of muscle, but if they have the same height and weight they will have the same BMI. It is therefore possible that one person may be extremely fit and have a BMI in the obese class, and yet another person may rather flabby and unfit and yet not be obese. A number of alternative metrics have been proposed as alternatives to BMI, including the waist to height ratio, waist to weight ratio, the Surface-based Body Shape Index and others.

However, despite evidence that some of these alternative measures capture clinically relevant details and actually correlate well to health outcomes, the BMI remains embedded in the health research arena. What this means is that in the following discussion on obesity and underweight the data that has been collected and analysed is largely structured around these BMI categories. If you are an individual who has a lot of muscle mass, an athlete for example, but who has an 'obese' or 'overweight' BMI score then it is less likely that the results will be relevant to you.

In terms of obesity as a risk factor for developing cancer in the first place the strongest evidence is in some hormonally-driven cancers, particularly advanced prostate and endometrial cancers, and in kidney and oesophageal cancers. There is also some evidence of risk for colorectal, post-menopausal breast and pancreatic cancer. In one well-known study it was estimated that:

*Excess body weight is the third most common avoidable cause of cancer in the UK, estimated to be responsible for 5.5% of cancers in 2010 (4.1% in men, 6.9% in women)* [26]

According to this same study, the four most important modifiable risk factors for cancer in the UK are tobacco (first by some considerable margin), diet, obesity and alcohol intake.

What influence does weight have on prognosis once cancer has been diagnosed? A number of studies have looked at the influence of body weight on overall survival and/or recurrence rates, and the findings have generally been consistent. Obesity, especially severe obesity, has an adverse effect on survival independent of other factors – in colorectal cancer [27], advanced breast cancer (especially in the post-menopausal [28]), endometrial cancers [29] and so on. The data is not unequivocal and there are some studies which fail to show a strong relationship. There are also some studies which show that being severely underweight is a significant risk factor in cancer-related mortality [30].

There are sound biological reasons to explain why being severely overweight or underweight might have negative impacts on cancer. The first is that both extremes of weight are associated with an increased level of oxidative stress – this is related to rates of chronic inflammation. While the relationship between chronic inflammation and obesity is well-known, there is also some evidence that it exists in severely underweight people too [31]. Chronic inflammation and oxidative stress are known drivers of cancer initiation and progression – and they are implicated in a wide range of other health conditions, including type II diabetes.

Reducing levels of oxidative stress and inflammation is therefore a good strategy to adopt. Diet can certainly help here – but just as important is physical activity. While exercise is not a topic covered in this chapter, it is covered in more detail on the chapter on stress and cancer, it really should be part of any life-style change you adopt in relation to cancer. Based on all of the above we can conclude that diet can have an influence on cancer risks and on long-term outcomes. Maintaining a healthy weight – which means reducing weight if you are obese, or gaining weight if you are severely underweight – is important. And changing your diet so that it is more 'anti-inflammatory' may help, both in weight loss/gain, and also in reducing the levels of oxidative stress which are implicated in poorer outcomes.

## An anti-inflammatory diet

What does an anti-inflammatory diet look like, and what evidence is there to support it? Probably the most detailed research on this has come from a group of researchers from the USA who have developed a Dietary Inflammatory Index (DII) [32]. This was based on a very detailed review of the data on the impacts of different foods and nutrients on a range of inflammatory markers, with different foods and nutrients given a score based on the evidence (with human data weighted more heavily than animal data). This process produced a score for a range of foods and nutrients, which could then be used to work out an inflammatory index based on a person's diet. This was then tested by comparing the inflammatory index with a measure of CRP (C-reactive protein, a common inflammatory marker in the blood) for around six hundred individuals over the course of a year. Analysis showed that changes in the inflammatory index, based on changes in the diet, were tracked closely by changes in the CRP score – that is, those people who switched to a more anti-inflammatory diet showed reductions in the blood levels of CRP.

The DII has since been used to look at the diet of different populations and a range of health outcomes, including cancer and cardiovascular disease. One good example is based on data from the Iowa

Women's Study, which has tracked around 34700 women between the ages of 55 and 69 since 1986 [33]. Analysis showed that a higher DII score was associated with an increased risk of developing colorectal cancer. Other work has shown a relationship with endometrial or liver cancers also. One large study, by the same team of researchers found an increased risk of all-cause and cancer-related mortality for those with the highest DII versus the lowest [34].

What are the components of an anti-inflammatory diet according to the DII?

Things to include are:

- Vegetables, including but not limited to, green leafy veg
- Dairy
- Fish and seafood
- Fruit
- Nuts
- Pulses
- Red wine
- Tea
- Eggs
- Poultry

Things which are not good:

- Fried foods (including chips)

- Beer and spirits
- High-sugar drinks
- Processed foods

In general the dietary pattern is close to what is called a Mediterranean diet (MedDiet), and in fact one recent meta-analysis that pooled the data from more than 50 other studies reported a significant positive effect of adherence to a Mediterranean diet across a wide range of cancer types [35]. The medical literature on this form of diet is huge and extends practically across all major health issues, from aging to obesity to heart disease to cancer. Of course there is an issue in that there are varying definitions for what constitutes the MedDiet – and for those who are interested there is even an academic paper that has reviewed the multiple definitions and summarised the results for us [36]. A handy summary table is included in the paper, which is reproduced below:

Table 1. Comparison of dietary recommendations for three Mediterranean diet pyramids.

| Foods | Oldway's Preservation and Trust (2009) [21] | Mediterranean Diet Foundation (2011) [5] | 1999 Greek Dietary Guidelines (1999) [22] [1] |
|---|---|---|---|
| Olive oil | Every meal | Every meal | Main added lipid |
| Vegetables | Every meal | ≥2 serves every meal | 6 serves daily |
| Fruits | Every meal | 1–2 serves every meal | 3 serves daily |
| Breads and cereals | Every meal | 1–2 serves every meal | 8 serves daily |
| Legumes | Every meal | ≥2 serves weekly | 3–4 serves weekly |
| Nuts | Every meal | 1–2 serves daily | 3–4 serves weekly |
| Fish/Seafood | Often, at least two times per week | ≥2 serves weekly | 5–6 servings weekly |
| Eggs | Moderate portions, daily to weekly | 2–4 serves weekly | 3 servings weekly |
| Poultry | Moderate portions, daily to weekly | 2 serves weekly | 4 servings weekly |
| Dairy foods | Moderate portions, daily to weekly | 2 serves daily | 2 serves daily |
| Red meat | Less often | <2 serves/week | 4 servings monthly |
| Sweets | Less often | <2 serves/week | 3 servings weekly |
| Red wine | In moderation | In moderation and respecting social beliefs | Daily in moderation |

[1] Serving sizes specified as: 25 g bread, 100 g potato, 50–60 g cooked pasta, 100 g vegetables, 80 g apple, 60 g banana, 100 g orange, 200 g melon, 30 g grapes, 1 cup milk or yoghurt, 1 egg, 60 g meat, 100 g cooked dry beans.

Note that an important aspect of this diet, particularly when it comes to weight loss, is that it is not a high-calorie diet. Excessive carbohydrates, including from sugary drinks, are not part of this diet. In terms of calories, there are variations depending on the definition, but in general the daily calorie intake is around 2200 – 2500 kCal per day, which is lower than the average daily intake in the UK and other advanced economies.

There are numerous online tools and plenty of books describing in more detail the MedDiet, including recipe books and checklists and so on. One free resource is available online at the Patient Info website (http://patient.info/pdf/9222.pdf).

Finally, it has to be stressed once again that diet is just one part of a bigger health picture, and there is increasing evidence that physical activity is of major importance, including for people suffering from cancer. It is no coincidence that the 5:2 diet, which combines a MedDiet with twice weekly low-carb days, is being combined with physical exercise in a number of clinical trials in breast cancer.

## Concluding remarks

While this chapter has looked at a lot of data and covered a variety of topics, the emphasis has largely been on 'hard science' and data that addresses a number of commonly held beliefs about diet and cancer. However, there is an altogether different dimension which has been barely touched upon and that is the social and psychological factors involved in food and drink. Diet is much more than a collection of nutrients and the biological effects of metabolism.

One of the most distressing aspects of a cancer diagnosis is the sudden loss of autonomy that is often experienced. Decisions are made by oncologists, surgeons, radiographers and a vast array of medical professionals. These decisions extend not just to big decisions about prognosis or treatments, but sometimes down to small decisions which are presented as a *fait accompli*. For some people it feels as though they have been reduced to a set of symptoms to be managed – they are no longer a person with cancer but a patient or an oncological case. Taking control of diet becomes, therefore, a means to assert some autonomy and control. While you may not be able to control what drugs you are treated with, or when your radiotherapy is scheduled or the dates of your scans, you can control what it is you eat and when. This retained sense of autonomy is enormously important to quality of life. Simply put this is something that really matters.

Over and above that sense of self, there is another role that diet can play and that is a social role. The sharing of food is an intrinsic part of being human. In every culture on the planet eating with others is important. And that is no less so when it comes to cancer. Enjoying meals with friends and family can have huge effects on the stress of dealing with the illness. Some people take the time to brush up on cooking skills, or to learn to cook new recipes or explore new ingredients. They take the time to cook rather than just throw something into the microwave. Here again there are positive effects independent of the specific foods and nutrients being consumed.

There are of course very physical effects that arise from these positive food and diet changes in terms of stress reduction. We return to the topic of stress and cancer in a later chapter, but for now suffice it to say that reducing levels of stress is an important issue for cancer patients. Diet can play a key part in this, both through the direct effects of anti-inflammatory diets, such as the MedDiet, and also in the indirect way that building a new relationship with food can have.

Finally, it is important to think of diet in a broader context that encompasses other aspects of lifestyle, including physical activity, exercise, sleep and stress management.

## Summary

- There is a huge amount that we don't understand about diet in general, not just about cancer and diet – keep in mind this uncertainty when you hear people talking as though cancer can be cured by diet alone
- There is no evidence for positive health effects from eating organic food, including organically reared meat. You may gain more positive effects from growing your own produce – gardening is good for you!
- While it is true that cancer cells may be addicted to glucose, due to what is known as the Warburg Effect, tumours are adaptable

and respond to nutrient availability in different ways. Low-carb diets may be helpful, particularly for people with weight issues or high levels of blood sugar

- Intermittent fasting may be helpful for cancer patients undergoing chemotherapy. However care has to be taken to avoid a catastrophic loss of weight
- Alkalising diets are often sold as cancer cures but there is very little evidence that they have any effect whatsoever
- There is little evidence to support the idea that dairy produce causes cancer or is associated with poorer cancer outcomes. There is some evidence that dairy yoghurts may have positive effects on the immune system
- There is little evidence to support the idea that meat consumption causes cancer, particularly when the intake is moderate. Some scare stories exaggerate the excess cancer risk associated with processed or red meat
- Moderate alcohol intake is associated with slightly improved overall mortality – primarily due to improved cardiovascular outcomes. However the evidence in cancer is mixed, but an occasional drink, particularly of red wine, may be beneficial
- Many dietary ingredients are sold as 'super-foods', but while there is evidence from test tube that specific foods have anti-cancer

properties when purified, there is little evidence that any single food has a significant effect in cancer

- Extreme weight (both obesity and extreme underweight) are associated with poorer health – in part this may be due to excessive amounts of oxidative stress or chronic inflammation
- Anti-inflammatory diets are associated with positive health and a reduced risk of a number of different cancer types. This type of diet is close to what is termed the Mediterranean diet

# References

1  Sinatra ST, Teter BB, Bowden J, Houston MC and Martinez-Gonzalez M a (2014) **The saturated fat, cholesterol, and statin controversy a commentary.** *Journal of the American College of Nutrition*, **33**(1), pp. 79–88.

2  Ramsden CE, Zamora D, Majchrzak-Hong S, Faurot KR, et al. (2016) **Re-evaluation of the traditional diet-heart hypothesis: analysis of recovered data from Minnesota Coronary Experiment (1968-73).** *BMJ (Clinical research ed.)*, **353**, p. i1246.

3    Virtanen JK, Mursu J, Virtanen HEK, Fogelholm M, et al. (2016) **Associations of egg and cholesterol intakes with carotid intima-media thickness and risk of incident coronary artery disease according to apolipoprotein e phenotype in men: The Kuopio Ischaemic Heart Disease Risk Factor Study**. *American Journal of Clinical Nutrition*, **103**(3), pp. 895–901.

4    USDA (2012) **2010 – 2011 Pilot Study Pesticide Residue Testing of Organic Produce**,

5    Hernández ÁR, Boada LD, Mendoza Z, Ruiz-Suárez N, et al. (2015) **Consumption of organic meat does not diminish the carcinogenic potential associated with the intake of persistent organic pollutants (POPs)**. *Environmental science and pollution research international*.

6    Smith-Spangler C, Brandeau ML, Hunter GE, Bavinger JC, et al. (2012) **Are organic foods safer or healthier than conventional alternatives?: a systematic review**. *Annals of internal medicine*, **157**(5), pp. 348–66.

7    Bradbury KE, Balkwill A, Spencer E a, Roddam A, et al. (2014) **Organic food**

consumption and the incidence of cancer in a large prospective study of women in the United Kingdom. *British Journal of Cancer*, **110**(9), pp. 2321–6.

8    Levêque-Morlais N, Tual S, Clin B, Adjemian A, et al. (2015) **The AGRIculture and CANcer (AGRICAN) cohort study: enrollment and causes of death for the 2005-2009 period.** *International archives of occupational and environmental health*, **88**(1), pp. 61–73.

9    Lemarchand C, Tual S, Boulanger M, Levêque-Morlais N, et al. (2016) **Prostate cancer risk among French farmers in the AGRICAN cohort.** *Scandinavian journal of work, environment & health*, **42**(2), pp. 144–52.

10   Blair CK, Madan-Swain A, Locher JL, Desmond RA, et al. (2013) **Harvest for health gardening intervention feasibility study in cancer survivors.** *Acta oncologica (Stockholm, Sweden)*, **52**(6), pp. 1110–8.

11   Woolf EC and Scheck AC (2014) **The Ketogenic Diet for the Treatment of Malignant Glioma.** *Journal of lipid research*, pp. 1–19.

12    Bonuccelli G, Whitaker-Menezes D, Castello-Cros R, Pavlides S, et al. (2010) **The reverse Warburg effect: glycolysis inhibitors prevent the tumor promoting effects of caveolin-1 deficient cancer associated fibroblasts.** *Cell cycle (Georgetown, Tex.)*, **9**(10), pp. 1960–71.

13    Raffaghello L, Lee C, Safdie FM, Wei M, et al. (2008) **Starvation-dependent differential stress resistance protects normal but not cancer cells against high-dose chemotherapy.** *Proceedings of the National Academy of Sciences of the United States of America*, **105**(24), pp. 8215–20.

14    Cheng CW, Adams GB, Perin L, Wei M, et al. (2014) **Prolonged fasting reduces IGF-1/PKA to promote hematopoietic-stem-cell-based regeneration and reverse immunosuppression.** *Cell Stem Cell*, **14**(6), pp. 810–823.

15    Safdie FM, Dorff T, Quinn D, Fontana L, et al. (2009) **Fasting and cancer treatment in humans: A case series report.** *Aging*, **1**(12), pp. 988–1007.

16    de Groot S, Vreeswijk MPG, Welters MJP, Gravesteijn G, et al. (2015) **The effects of**

short-term fasting on tolerance to (neo) adjuvant chemotherapy in HER2-negative breast cancer patients: a randomized pilot study.** *BMC cancer*, **15**(1), p. 652.

17    Berrigan D, Perkins SN, Haines DC and Hursting SD (2002) **Adult-onset calorie restriction and fasting delay spontaneous tumorigenesis in p53-deficient mice.** *Carcinogenesis*, **23**(5), pp. 817–22.

18    Chan DSM, Lau R, Aune D, Vieira R, et al. (2011) **Red and processed meat and colorectal cancer incidence: meta-analysis of prospective studies.** *PloS one*, **6**(6), p. e20456.

19    Appleby PN, Crowe FL, Bradbury KE, Travis RC and Key TJ (2015) **Mortality in vegetarians and comparable nonvegetarians in the United Kingdom**. *American Journal of Clinical Nutrition*, p. ajcn.115.119461–.

20    Chao C, Haque R, Caan BJ, Poon K-YT, et al. (2010) **Red wine consumption not associated with reduced risk of colorectal cancer.** *Nutrition and cancer*, **62**(6), pp. 849–55.

21    Chao C, Haque R, Van Den Eeden SK, Caan BJ, et al. (2010) **Red wine consumption and risk of prostate cancer: the California men's health study.** *International journal of cancer*, **126**(1), pp. 171–9.

22    Cook LS, Leung ACY, Swenerton K, Gallagher RP, et al. (2016) **Adult lifetime alcohol consumption and invasive epithelial ovarian cancer risk in a population-based case-control study.** *Gynecologic oncology*, **140**(2), pp. 277–84.

23    Toledo E, Salas-Salvadó J, Donat-Vargas C, Buil-Cosiales P, et al. (2015) **Mediterranean Diet and Invasive Breast Cancer Risk Among Women at High Cardiovascular Risk in the PREDIMED Trial: A Randomized Clinical Trial.** *JAMA internal medicine*, **175**(11), pp. 1752–60.

24    Thomas R, Williams M, Sharma H, Chaudry A and Bellamy P (2014) **A double-blind, placebo-controlled randomised trial evaluating the effect of a polyphenol-rich whole food supplement on PSA progression in men with prostate cancer--the U.K. NCRN Pomi-T study.** *Prostate cancer and prostatic diseases*, **17**(2), pp. 180–6.

25    Wu L, Wang Z, Zhu J, Murad AL, et al. (2015) **Nut consumption and risk of cancer and type 2 diabetes: a systematic review and meta-analysis.** *Nutrition reviews*, **73**(7), pp. 409–25.

26    Parkin DM, Boyd L and Walker LC (2011) **16. The fraction of cancer attributable to lifestyle and environmental factors in the UK in 2010.** *British journal of cancer*, **105 Suppl** , pp. S77–81.

27    Daniel CR, Shu X, Ye Y, Gu J, et al. (2016) **Severe obesity prior to diagnosis limits survival in colorectal cancer patients evaluated at a large cancer centre.** *British journal of cancer*, **114**(1), pp. 103–9.

28    Iwase T, Sangai T, Nagashima T, Sakakibara M, et al. (2016) **Impact of body fat distribution on neoadjuvant chemotherapy outcomes in advanced breast cancer patients.** *Cancer medicine*, **5**(1), pp. 41–8.

29    Secord AA, Hasselblad V, Von Gruenigen VE, Gehrig PA, et al. (2016) **Body mass index and mortality in endometrial cancer: A systematic review and meta-analysis.** *Gynecologic oncology*, **140**(1), pp. 184–90.

30    Reichle K, Peter RS, Concin H and Nagel G (2015) **Associations of pre-diagnostic body mass index with overall and cancer-specific mortality in a large Austrian cohort.** *Cancer causes & control: CCC*, **26**(11), pp. 1643–52.

31    Mizoue T, Tokunaga S, Kasai H, Kawai K, et al. (2007) **Body mass index and oxidative DNA damage: A longitudinal study.** *Cancer Science*, **98**(8), pp. 1254–1258.

32    Cavicchia PP, Steck SE, Hurley TG, Hussey JR, et al. (2009) **A new dietary inflammatory index predicts interval changes in serum high-sensitivity C-reactive protein.** *The Journal of nutrition*, **139**(12), pp. 2365–72.

33    Shivappa N, Prizment AE, Blair CK, Jacobs DR, et al. (2014) **Dietary Inflammatory Index and Risk of Colorectal Cancer in the Iowa Women's Health Study.** *Cancer epidemiology, biomarkers & prevention: a publication of the American Association for Cancer Research, cosponsored by the American Society of Preventive Oncology*, **23**(11), pp. 2383–92.

34    Shivappa N, Steck SE, Hussey JR, Ma Y and

Hebert JR (2015) **Inflammatory potential of diet and all-cause, cardiovascular, and cancer mortality in National Health and Nutrition Examination Survey III Study.** *European journal of nutrition.*

35    Schwingshackl L and Hoffmann G (2015) **Adherence to Mediterranean diet and risk of cancer: an updated systematic review and meta-analysis of observational studies.** *Cancer medicine*, **4**(12), pp. 1933–47.

36    Davis C, Bryan J, Hodgson J and Murphy K (2015) **Definition of the Mediterranean Diet; a Literature Review.** *Nutrients*, **7**(11), pp. 9139–53.

# Cancer and the Media

## Introduction

It is impossible to avoid the topic of cancer in the mass media – from 'old' media such as newspapers and print magazines to web sites, blogs and social media platforms. Stories range from news on celebrities who have been diagnosed with the disease, to breathless stories of exciting new breakthroughs to political discussions around the costs or the availability of the latest generation of anticancer drugs. At the best of times this profusion of stories can be confusing, but for a cancer patient or carer looking at the news these issues can be more urgent. For example, does a story about a new treatment stand up to scrutiny? Is this really a new treatment or just an idea about a treatment that may or may not be developed in the future? Or perhaps there is a story that a particular food is associated with preventing cancer – is there really evidence for this, and if so what does it mean in the context of someone already diagnosed with the disease?

This chapter will look at a number of common themes that recur frequently in how the media portray cancer research and provide some guidelines to help interpret the evidence.

## Substance *X* Cures Cancer

A very common story that appears in the press and on the internet is one in which a particular substance cures cancer. A number of recent examples include a curry spice called turmeric, cannabis oil, oxygen, avocados, a type of Australian berry and coffee. It may sometimes seem that there are so many 'cures' out there that it's a wonder anyone ever suffers from the disease. There have even been occasions when the same popular newspaper has reported on two different cures on the same day! The examples listed are just a small sample from the many that crop up every day. Some, like turmeric or cannabis, recur frequently, whereas some of the others only turn up once and then disappear without trace.

What these stories have in common is the idea that a single substance can cure cancer. The headlines are always framed in those terms. The story isn't about a treatment as such; it's about a particular ingredient or medicinal agent – often not a drug but a food, herb, spice or nutraceutical (food-derived product which has medicinal properties, for example certain vitamins) – which can cure cancer.

While the stories may vary in the detail there are a number of common themes which emerge from them. One set of stories in this category is based on scientific research of one type or another. Broadly speaking this type of story is reporting on scientific data or the output of a piece of research. In contrast another type of 'substance cures cancer' story is reporting on a personal anecdote – for example the story of a person who has cured him or herself of cancer by taking the given substance. And a final type of story that is more common on the internet than in mainstream press is the conspiracy theory. Here the story is that a given substance with curative powers is actively being suppressed by the medical profession or the drug companies. Let's look at each of these types of story in turn.

## *Research*

Very few of the research-based stories will actually be about treating people with cancer. Instead that stunning headline will usually give way to more detail in which it is revealed that the given substance has been shown to kill cancer cells in a test tube. Sometimes there may even be talk of using the substance in mice or rats and that these have responded well to the treatment. Generally the curing cancer bit applies rather more to the test tube than the animals, though there are times when there are good results in animals too. However, there is a huge world of difference between what happens in a test tube or petri dish in which it is rather easy to kill cancer cells and what happens in an animal. Of course there is an even bigger jump from specially bred lab mice to people.

The exciting headlines are of course down to the journalists who write the stories rather than the scientists carrying out the experiments. Or, as is increasingly common, the exciting headlines are from a public relations agency working for the university or research institute where the research was carried out. It might even originate from a charity or not for profit organisation that funded the research. The aim in all these cases is to generate some media publicity in the hope that it will help raise the profile of the organisation and perhaps bring in additional future funding. But whether it's the journalists or the PR people who wrote the press release that went to the journalists, the result is the same – a set of headlines which promise more than they can deliver.

That said, for anyone who wants to explore a particular story further there are a number of steps which can be taken. The first is simply to note down the names of the scientists who are reported to have performed the work and then to use an online scientific database or search engine, such as PubMed or Google Scholar, to find the original research papers that report the results of the research. In some cases the original press release, which will often be available on a university website, will contain a link to the original paper. The original paper will have the full details of the research which has been distilled down to a couple of breathless paragraphs for the mass media. In addition, the paper or the university web site will also have a contact email address so that it is possible to contact the researchers directly should you want to.

## *Personal Anecdote*

In contrast to the research story, the personal anecdote does not pretend to be based on scientific research, though in some cases there will be an attempt to explain some part of the story in what sound like scientific terms. In general terms the narrative will be along the lines of a person who either refused treatment or who had reached the end of the line as regards standard treatments and had taken whatever the magic substance is and then staged a stunning recovery. In many such stories the recovery will reported as a 'cure' – much to the amazement of the doctors who had given up all hope. This is to all intents and purposes the story of a miracle and one which we all want to believe, especially if we are in dire straits or supporting a loved one facing a grim prognosis.

Is there anything that we can sensibly say about such fantastic stories? Can we credit any such stories with a grain of truth? Does it mean that we should follow suit and also take whatever the magic substance was?

The first thing to point out is that there are genuine cases of fantastic and unexpected recoveries. These are often referred to as *spontaneous remissions* in the medical literature. They do exist but they are incredibly rare. It is believed that these events are associated with the immune system suddenly kicking in and ridding the body of cancer. Indeed, much scientific research is about trying to do exactly that. However, many of the stories in the press do not fit with this type of event – many cases of spontaneous remission are associated with infections, fever and flu-like symptoms. There are some cases reported in the medical literature where there are sustained remissions brought about by unorthodox treatments – for example long-term stable disease associated with repurposed drugs such as antifungal drugs. But again these differ from the stories in the press in that the treatment is not classed as a 'cure' and there is normally evidence from medical records to back up the claims being made. In the personal anecdotes reported in the press there is generally no corroborating evidence.

Furthermore, if you read between the lines you will often see that the person was taking a number of other substances at the same time. Whereas the headlines might claim that it was substance X, it turns out that the person was also undergoing some form of standard treatment – for example maintenance therapy or metronomic chemotherapy (covered in a separate chapter) – as well as a number of other vitamins, minerals, herbs and so on.

At the end of the day even if we are generous and do not dismiss the story as more fiction than fact, what can we usefully gain from it? At most, it might pique an interest in substance X and we can investigate the scientific research on that substance.

*Conspiracy Theory*

The final version of 'substance X cures cancer' is the idea of a conspiracy theory – of which there are many to choose from. As with the previous examples, the magic substance varies but the underlying narrative is the same. The basic plot is simple – a cancer cure exists that is safe and cheap but which threatens the powers that be. Therefore the secret has been suppressed and millions of patients are being denied the chance for a cure. Who is running this conspiracy? Governments, the medical profession and the big drugs companies. Why? Because a cure that is cheap and safe threatens the profits of the drug companies, who pay a fortune to governments in the form of taxes, and threatens the livelihood of the doctors who treat all these cancer patients. It's a simple idea that is embellished with all kinds of details and additional elements and, unfortunately, repeated on countless websites and blogs.

Many of the conspiracy theories are laced with scientific sounding explanations – in some cases there may even be some real science embedded in amongst the fiction. But at the end of the day there is nothing of value to be gained from these stories. Firstly, the sad fact is that there is no secret cure. In every case that is brought up – from cannabis oil to GcMAF to anti-neoplastons and beyond – the scientific evidence is simply not there. In some cases the 'story' depends on an explanation of what cancer is and how it develops that does not match the complex reality of the disease. For example there is no evidence that cancer is a fungus that can be cured by the direct application of sodium bicarbonate – a story that gained quite a bit of publicity in some quarters for a while.

The fact is that if someone did come up with a cure for a cancer, even one that only worked for a subset of cancers, there is no way that the information could be kept secret. No drugs company could keep it quiet

– aside from the fear that someone would find out and cause a massive scandal – there would be the danger that someone else would discover the same thing and therefore be able to claim the scientific credit and the financial rewards. The biggest rewards are for being the first with a discovery. Furthermore, for this kind of conspiracy to be successful it would need thousands upon thousands of individuals to take part in hiding the truth.

Finally, it has to be said that in many cases the people making the strongest case for a conspiracy are those who are profiting directly by selling something. In some cases it might be a book or video about the conspiracy and the secret cure, in other cases it's someone selling the so-called cure – from people selling cannabis oil to those who are raking in millions selling GcMAF to desperate people, while all the time claiming doctors and researchers are driven entirely by greed.

## Cancer Is Caused By X

Another very common story in media is the 'cause of cancer' story. The starting point for many of these stories is often a new piece of research, particularly if the story is in the news or in the mass media. There is also a subset of stories which appear more frequently on small websites and blogs but which are closer to the conspiracy theory view of the world than the science-based view. In either case it may sometimes appear to the reader that according to some parts of the media there are just as many causes as there are probable cures!

We can group the 'causes' into a number of popular categories: food and drink, lifestyle, toxins and technology. Let's look at each of these in turn.

### *Food and Drink*

This a common theme in many media reports on cancer. The typical story will run along the lines of 'doctors say that eating (or drinking) $X$ causes cancer'. The range of items that have been listed in recent years includes red meat, alcohol, rice, peanuts, fats, refined sugars and more. The source for these stories normally comes from two types of scientific study.

The first is what is called an epidemiological study in which researchers analyse data for large populations in a bid to try and find associations between the incidence of disease and certain behaviours. In this type of study the scientists might look at several thousand people and then see if those who developed cancer were more or less likely to eat or drink a certain item. Usually they will start with an idea that there might be a link – for example because it is known that a type of fungus called aflatoxin can cause cancer and it is known to infect peanuts. Alternatively they might be looking at two populations and will want to see why one set is more prone to cancer than another set. In any case these epidemiological studies depend on large populations to detect any associations. However such studies suffer from some serious weaknesses. In the first case there are often confounding variables involved. For example it might be that people who consume a lot of peanuts are also people who spend a lot of time in bars and have a higher alcohol intake, or else they engage in behaviours that are less healthy than non-peanut consumers. Secondly, it is often the case that these studies can prove association but not causation – for example there is an association between sun-burn and ice cream consumption, but that doesn't mean that ice cream causes sun-burn.

A second type of scientific study related to this story is the test tube study in which cells in a test tube or petri dish are exposed to high concentrations of the food or drink in question and then the cells show signs of genetic damage which might cause cancer. A variation on this type of study is to feed specially bred laboratory mice a diet that is high in the food or drink and then see how many of them develop cancer. In many cases these are mice which are designed to develop cancers relatively easily. As with the cancer cures stories, there is a world of difference between what goes on in a test tube or lab mouse and what goes on in humans. In fact there's a world of difference between what goes on in these lab mice and in their cousins in the wild.

Regardless of the origin of these stories they will both be reported with alarming headlines in the press. In particular much will be made of the increases in risk associated with consumption of the guilty item. The vast majority of reports will use what is called the *relative risk* – which is also often the metric that the epidemiologists themselves will use, so it is not just the fault of journalists. The problem with relative risk is that it's actually not that useful a measure in real life. If you are told that eating something doubles your risk of developing oesophageal cancer compared to not eating it then that's a scary story. But if your risk is actually one in a million then doubling it to two in a million is not such a scare after all.

We should also mention the fact that there are a number of common misconceptions about the dietary influence on cancer. The first is the idea that pesticides in food cause cancer, and that therefore eating organic food is a healthier option. The evidence for this assertion does not exist – as explained in the chapter on cancer and diet. The fact is that there is no evidence for a health benefit in eating organic produce, including no evidence of a protective effect against cancer. Similarly there are some people who will claim that dairy produce can cause hormonally linked cancers, particularly breast cancer. Again there is no evidence to back up this claim – in fact there is evidence the other way to show that some of the fats in dairy are protective against cancer.

The bottom line is that we actually have a pretty good idea of what the main causes of cancer are: smoking, certain infections (Helicobactor, HPV, Hepatitis B etc), genetic predispositions (Li Fraumeni Syndrome, BRCA1/BRCA2, Lynch Syndrome), aging and so on. There is some evidence that some types of diet are less healthy than others, and we know that obesity raises cancer risk too. But on the whole many of the stories in the press, even though they are based on scientific reports, are a lot less scary than the headlines would suggest.

*Lifestyle*
In this category we have stories associated with particular behaviours rather than food and drink. Examples include smoking, exercise, sleep patterns, psychological stress and so on. As with the previous section, there are new stories appearing in the press

constantly, as well as frequent references to old stories in light of new evidence. However, in contrast to food and diet, which are somewhat difficult to pin down, there really are some lifestyle factors which are very strongly associated with an increased risk of cancer.

As before, many of the news stories are connected with newly published research. Many of the comments which applied to epidemiological studies with diet also apply to lifestyle factors. It's hard to unravel cause and effect, and of course there is always the risk of *confounding variables* and factors which simply do not appear in the data. To go back to our correlation between sun-burn and ice cream, one obvious confounding factor is temperature – hot, sunny days increase the risk of sun-burn and increase the consumption of ice cream.

That said, one of the biggest cancer risk factors is definitely related to lifestyle, and that is smoking. Where many of the factors reported in the press have limited evidence for them, there is strong evidence for the risks of smoking – from laboratory experiments which show the effects of smoking at the molecular level to animal experiments to very strong epidemiological data.

Other risk factors with strong evidence are an association with obesity, lack of exercise, shift work and excessive stress. And, as with smoking, there is a range of different types of evidence that we can draw on to support these links. Scientists have an idea of the mechanisms at work, we have animal evidence and there is evidence from human populations that we can draw on.

## Technology

Given the apparent increases in worldwide cancer incidence it is natural that people look for the underlying causes. In addition to diet and lifestyle many people have also looked at some of the technological advances of recent years to see if they have had an impact on cancer incidence. Unfortunately this is another area where the press can get carried away with scary headlines based on incredibly weak levels of evidence. And, even more unfortunate this is one of the areas where the internet is also rife with conspiracy theories and misinformation.

One of the biggest technological advances of recent decades has been the explosion of mobile communications technology – from mobile phones onwards. It would appear that this increase in prevalence of mobile technology has coincided with an increase in worldwide cancer rates. There are many people, including a few scientists, who believe that this is no accident. This is an area where there has been intense research activity and to date there is no clear picture that has emerged.

The biggest fear has been that mobile phone technology is linked to an increase in brain tumours but again there is no clear evidence that this is the case. Detailed analysis shows that there has been no increase in the rate of brain tumours in the population. Nor is there a clear indication that users of mobile technology are over-represented in the numbers – although some researchers have claimed to see a small relationship between brain tumour incidence and the *heaviest* users of mobile and cordless phones. Currently even this link is open to dispute. A very thorough recent study from Australia that looked at the connection between mobile phones and brain tumours, using almost thirty years of data, concluded that there was no increased risk [1].

The most that can be said is that it is possible that excessive mobile phone use might be carcinogenic, and that therefore caution has to be exercised by those who are very, very heavy users. However, this measured and cautious approach is not apparent in the media, where there are frequent alarmist stories about mobile phones causing cancer. Still worse are some of the wild claims made by conspiracy theorists on the wilder shores of the internet. There are some who claim that nearly all forms of electromagnetic technology are the cause of cancer – and in this they include not just mobile phones but cordless phones, microwave cookers, televisions, wi-fi networks, pylons and electricity distribution networks, RFID devices in supermarkets and more. The tone of many of these sites encourages paranoia and a distrust of many benign and useful technologies.

What is worse is that some of the people making these claims also sell devices which they claim can 'shield' users from 'harmful rays' that would otherwise cause cancer. Many of these devices are both incredibly expensive and invasive and disruptive of normal life. The danger is that vulnerable people battling with cancer might be fooled by the apparent scientific tone of some of these articles. For people struggling with the stress of a cancer diagnosis and having to go through the rigours of treatment, the paranoia induced by these websites can only add to the pressure. Additionally the financial investment required to buy these expensive devices can be quite considerable – again at a time when resources are likely to be scarce. People who deliberately stoke up a fear of technology in order to make money from cancer patients are little different from those who peddle fake cures in order to make vast profits from other people's misery.

While this section has focused on mobile technologies, these are by no means the only forms of technology that some people blame as the cause of cancer. There is frequent mention of various forms of environmental toxin or sources of pollution, water fluoridisation, plastics and endocrine disruptive chemicals and more. In nearly all cases there is more fiction than fact involved – and normally the more hysterical the tone of the article the less there is in the way of credible evidence of cause and effect.

## Substance *X* Prevents Cancer

The final theme in this survey of common cancer-related stories in the media is that class of stories in which a given substance, often but not always a food item, can prevent cancer occurring in the first place. In many respects this has features in common with the 'substance *X* cures cancer' stories, and in fact many of the same items appear in both. Common examples include certain spices (curcumin, from the curry spice turmeric for example), berries, green tea, soya, vitamin C, organic fruit and vegetables and more. Other non-food items include exercise, meditation and stress reduction, proper sleep and so on.

As before, the stories are derived from many sources, usually being linked to a newly published piece of scientific research. These will range from population studies to animal work or laboratory experiments using cell cultures. As with all research the quality will vary, and the weight we should place on such stories will vary accordingly. However, because these are stories about initial cancer prevention there is less urgency to them for readers of this book than stories about probable cures or treatments.

That said there are some closing remarks that are worth making. The first is that the causes of cancer are many and varied, even with people who have a genetic predisposition to the disease. Some people may smoke for decades and never develop cancer, others may enjoy a healthy diet and do plenty of exercise and still develop the disease at an early age. The danger is that some people become so convinced that they understand that certain diets or lifestyles cause cancer that they almost blame cancer patients for developing the disease in the first place. So, while it is interesting to know that cutting down on red meat or taking up regular exercise reduces overall risk, it does not mean that someone who enjoys a sedentary lifestyle and a good steak is at fault if they develop the disease.

## Summary

- The media, including the internet and social media, often carry extraordinary stories about cancer, particularly when it comes to reporting 'cancer cures'
- If a story sounds too good to be true then it's probably not true
- Many reported cures are based on personal anecdote and do not stand up to scrutiny
- The best response to these stories is to remain sceptical – and to use the examples in this chapter to categorise new stories as they appear in the press

## References

1    Chapman S, Azizi L, Luo Q and Sitas F (2016) **Has the incidence of brain cancer risen in Australia since the introduction of mobile phones 29 years ago?** *Cancer Epidemiology.*

# Understanding Clinical Trials

## Introduction

Clinical trials are the main way that new medical treatments and systems are tested in people. Each trial is designed to answer a very specific set of questions and understanding these questions, and how the trial intends to answer them, is of fundamental importance if you are considering joining a trial. This chapter will look at how trials are constructed, what types of questions they are designed to answer and what factors are important both to the patient and to the doctors and scientists running the trials. While many trials, particularly in cancer, are testing drug treatments of different types, there are also trials that involve non-drug treatments such as surgery, radiotherapy, photodynamic therapy, ablation or new forms of imaging (for example new types of MRI or ultrasound scans). While many of the examples that follow are geared around drug trials, the same principles apply to the non-drug trials.

The starting point for any discussion of clinical trials is to establish what the primary aim of the trial is. For many patients with cancer the main interest is in clinical trials that are testing new treatments – both curative and non-curative (more on this difference later). However, there are also trials which are designed to look at specific characteristics of a disease – for example looking at special markers in the blood or genetic sampling of tumours. There are trials which are designed to look at social or psychological factors – for example to assess the support needs of cancer patients or to explore feelings of depression or anxiety. Other trials may be testing new scanning or diagnostic equipment – looking at how ultrasound scans can be used to diagnose breast cancer in addition to mammograms for example. Finally, there may be trials of cancer prevention strategies – diet or exercise or other life-style changes in high-risk groups.

While this article will look in more detail at treatment-related clinical trials, we should say a few words about these non-treatment trials. Improving our understanding of cancer is of huge importance and while the patients participating may not benefit directly from joining a trial looking at biomarkers (measurable substances in the blood or tissues that tell us about a disease or condition) or new diagnostic techniques, ultimately the knowledge gained will be of benefit to patients in the future. In particular, if we can diagnose cancer sooner, or become better at understanding which biomarkers are important to assessing the success or otherwise of treatment, the benefits to patients will be immense. Similarly, finding out if there are strategies to reduce cancer risks in high-risk groups, such as women with a family history of breast or ovarian cancer, will ultimately save lives. In many cases these non-treatment related clinical trials are carried out in parallel with existing treatments, diagnostics and scanning procedures and therefore have little impact on current practice. Assuming that there is little or no negative impact then joining these trials may be seen as part of 'doing your bit' for the good of society at large.

The actual process of searching for a trial and the practical issues involved in applying for participation are not covered in this chapter. The next chapter is devoted specifically to those kinds of issues. With that in mind the main focus here will be on learning more about the design and structure of treatment-related clinical trials.

## What is the treatment for?

Not all treatment-related trials are looking at potential new cures for cancer. Cancer is a complex set of diseases that can produce many different symptoms, including some that are painful and debilitating. Cancer treatments, particularly chemotherapy and radiotherapy, often cause nasty side effects, such as nausea, vomiting, hair loss and so on. These side effects can often be worse than the symptoms of the cancer itself. There is active research looking at ways of reducing these symptoms and side effects, mostly through the use of medicines, and these treatments need to be tested in clinical trials in just the same way that new curative treatments have to be.

More generally one way of thinking about treatment-related clinical trials is to separate them into curative and palliative treatments. Curative treatments aim at directly attacking the cancer in order to cure the disease completely – for example with drugs that are toxic to tumour cells, or which arm the immune system so that it can attack the tumours or which block specific chemical pathways that tumours need to survive.

Palliative treatments are aimed at addressing the quality of life issues through symptom reduction. Palliative treatments are not necessarily only used at late stages of disease, so to be referred to a trial of a palliative treatment does not mean that an oncologist is no longer treating a patient with curative intent. Some palliative treatments will seek to address those debilitating symptoms by attempting to reduce tumour size. Examples include radiotherapy, radio-frequency ablation, photodynamic therapy or cryoablation. In this situation the cancer is being attacked directly in order to shrink tumour size but the intention is primarily to exert local control of the disease rather than to affect a cure. In such a situation it is very important to be clear about the primary purpose of the treatment because it may be easy to be confused about what the treatment is attempting to achieve.

To be clear then, curative treatments aim at a cure, palliative treatments aim at symptom control. Palliative treatments are used at all stages of disease, but there are some palliative treatments which aim at local control of disease when there are no longer any curative options available.

## Clinical trial phases

Clinical trials come in all shapes and sizes, often depending on what stage in the process of development a treatment has progressed to. Typically trials are ranked by phase, with the earliest steps in the process being described as Phase 0 or Phase I and ending with Phase IV trials after a new treatment has become adopted in clinical practice. These different phases of trials are designed to find the answers to different questions. We can look at each of these in turn to understand the key features of them.

## Phase 0

Phase 0 trials are a relatively recent addition to the clinical trials process. These are very small trials designed to expedite the drug development process. They are explicitly designed to determine the pharmacological properties of a new drug. In other words these trials are designed to test whether a new drug reaches the cells it is supposed to target, how long the drug is present in the blood stream, what kind of toxicity it causes and so on. To achieve these a very small number of patients are used, typically fewer than 10 and they are treated for a short period (often for less than a week). The new drug is used at a very low dose, lower than the dose at which it will show any significant therapeutic effect. The drugs in Phase 0 trials have not normally been tested in people before, although there is pre-clinical evidence in animals to give some idea of safety and effect.

Assessment of the pharmacological properties of the new drug will typically involve blood tests, physical monitoring, scans and other procedures. It may also entail taking samples of tumour tissues or biopsies.

From a patient perspective there is no expectation whatsoever of a direct patient benefit from participation in a Phase 0 trial. However, there is much that can be learned about a new type of drug in such a trial, and the information can be used to speed up a development process that might otherwise take a number of years to bring these drugs to trials in humans. In terms of accelerating the development of new cancer drugs these Phase 0 trials are important, but patients taking part must be aware that they cannot gain therapeutic benefit from participation.

## Phase I

The Phase I trial is typically the first time that new drugs are tested at clinically relevant doses. Mostly Phase I trials are relatively small, both in terms of the number of patients and the duration of treatment that they undergo. The primary aims are normally to assess the kinds of toxicity (side effects) that result from the treatment, whether the drug or treatment gets to the cells that it is targeted at, how long the drug stays in the blood stream and so on. In many ways a Phase I trial is very like a Phase 0 trial except that the doses that are used are in what is believed to be a clinically relevant therapeutic range. It should be noted that in non-life-threatening diseases most patients in Phase I trials are healthy individuals, but this is not the case with cancer where many of the drugs are fairly toxic and may have significant side effects associated with them.

The drugs in Phase I trials are not necessarily new; some of them may have been used previously in other diseases or at radically different dosing schedules. In some cases a Phase I trial may investigate the combination of well-known drugs that have never been used together before, and there is a need to assess the safety and tolerability of the combination. Some Phase I trials may simply take existing cancer treatments and try them for the first time in a new cancer type or patient population.

Because toxicity and tolerability are key concerns of Phase I trials, patients participating in these trials are assessed frequently with blood tests, scans, biopsies and other relevant monitoring. A common pattern of these trials is the dose escalation trial where patients are recruited in batches, with the first batch starting at a low dose of the drug and subsequent batches receiving higher doses until a maximum tolerated dose has been achieved. While Phase I trials do treat some patients at clinically relevant doses, patients at the lowest doses may not receive a high enough dose to show any activity. Patients at later stages of a dose escalation trial may receive doses higher than the dose ultimately selected as the maximum tolerated dose.

Because the drugs being tested in many Phase I trials have not been proved to be effective, (or not effective in that particular type of cancer), many patients who take part will not benefit directly. While the trial will be looking for some evidence of efficacy, this is not normally the main outcome of these trials. The main intent of the Phase I trial is to prove the treatment has an acceptable safety profile, testing the ultimate effectiveness of the drug is normally something explored in later phases. That said there are some patients who do show some benefit from Phase I trials. However, most patients recruited to Phase I trials in oncology are those for whom there are no other clinical options open.

If you are a patient looking for a clinical trial it is not recommended that you start with a Phase I trial if later phase trials are available. Obviously if there are no other options available then a Phase I trial may be attractive. In assessing the decision whether to participate in the trial it is important to evaluate things carefully. For example, you would want to know how many other trials have used the drug; if it is a dose escalation trial you would want to know how many patients have previously been recruited; you would want to know what pre-clinical evidence exists (i.e. evidence from animal experiments); you would want to know what the research team already know about side effects and so on. This is not an easy decision to make and a discussion both with your oncologist and the trial team would normally take place.

## Phase II

In Phase II trials the main aim is to test a treatment for evidence of clinical effectiveness (often referred to as efficacy) rather than purely to investigate side effects or dosing. In the case of a Phase II drug trial the dose has normally been established in a previous Phase I trial, or else if it is a drug that is used in other forms of disease (including a different cancer type), then the dose will be based on current usage. This does not mean that there are no concerns about safety or side effects – typically a Phase II trial will include more patients than in a Phase I trial, and for a new drug additional side effects may occur that did not in the smaller trial. However, the main question that a Phase II trial is designed to answer is whether the treatment shows evidence that it works against disease.

There are a number of ways that you can test for evidence that a treatment is working, and thus there is a wide range of Phase II trial designs. In some trials the aim is just to treat all the patients with the drug or treatment and to record what happens – does the tumour shrink, are the side effects reduced, are patients in remission for a long period etc. In this kind of trial the patients are tracked, scanned, undergo blood tests and so on. How they do may be compared to patients who have had the same disease and staging and who were treated in the past – these are called *historical controls*.

Another form of Phase II trial may compare two groups of patients, those who receive the treatment and those who do not. Those that do not are called the *control group*. In some cases the control group do not receive any treatment; more often they receive the current standard treatment. Occasionally there are multiple sets of patients, with different groups receiving different doses or different treatments. The aim here is to gather data so that you can compare the effectiveness of a new treatment against one or more alternatives.

In some larger Phase II trials the control group may be treated with a dummy drug called a placebo. This is most often done in a trial which is randomised – which will be covered in a later section.

For patients looking for clinical trials Phase II trials are preferable to Phase I, but it is important to keep in mind that a Phase II trial has not yet established whether the treatment works or not. Obviously individual trials vary and some may be very speculative while others have a higher degree of knowledge associated with them. For example, a treatment that has shown some success in other cancers may be a more attractive option than a treatment that is completely new and has only just been through Phase I. A trial that is randomised and includes a group taking a placebo means there is a chance you will not get the new drug, whereas in a Phase II trial without a control group this is not the case. Finally, if there is data from previous trials, then take the time to investigate it. If you need help to interpret it then seek advice from your oncology team or look for additional help.

## Phase III

Phase III trials are normally the final phase of trial before a treatment becomes adopted as standard of care. As one would expect, a treatment would normally have successfully completed one or more Phase II trials before it can proceed to a Phase III trial. Typically these trials are much larger and normally include patients from multiple hospitals and clinics, often in multiple countries. Some larger Phase III trials will include thousands of patients. In part this is because a new treatment may only show marginal improvement over the existing standard of care, in which case you need to include more patients to ensure that the results are not simply down to chance.

As with the other phases of trial, safety and toxicity are closely monitored, even when there is a good safety profile established from the earlier trials. Because Phase III trials include a larger pool of patients there is still a chance that some rare side effects will manifest themselves for the first time.

Typically Phase III trials test the treatment against a control group receiving the standard of care treatment, and almost always in a randomised fashion.

While the Phase II trial will have shown that there is some evidence that the new treatment works, it is still possible that this was a statistical fluke and that the positive results are not replicated in the larger trial. The larger pool of patients will include patients from a wider range of ages, physical condition, disease staging and so on. A smaller trial will not match the variability in patient population that matches the real world; the Phase III trial is much more realistic in this sense.

While there may be more confidence that the Phase III treatment will work, having been through a number of earlier trials, there are still some things to keep in mind when assessing participation in such a trial. The first and most obvious is that randomisation may mean that you do not receive the new treatment. Secondly, it is important to assess the evidence established to date. For example the new treatment may offer increased progression free survival, but at the cost of significant side effects that negatively impact quality of life.

## Phase IV

After a drug or treatment has been through one or more Phase III trials and has been licensed, it may then become a standard treatment and be used on thousands of new patients. In this case it is still important to track the safety and efficacy of the treatment. This is more like long-term tracking of patient data rather than testing that has been performed in Phases I, II and III. Sometimes this process is called post-marketing surveillance rather than a Phase IV trial. In any case, this is not normally a process that a patient applies to join as the treatment itself is available direct from clinicians outside of a formal trial. However, it is important in that even the largest of Phase III trials will not treat the range and number of patients that a successful treatment will once it has been licensed. There have been some cases where Phase IV data has shown that some drugs do pose a risk to particular groups of patients.

## Mixed Phase Trials

In practice the neat distinctions between the different phases are not always adhered to. Some trials will not have a Phase attached to them – this is common for trials looking at tracking biomarkers, cancer prevention strategies, psychological interventions and so on. Sometimes early phase trials might be described as Pilot trials without necessarily specifying Phase I or Phase II. More commonly you will find that some trials combine phases, for example establishing a safe dose of a drug before moving straight into looking for evidence of efficacy, in other words a Phase I/II trial. In every case the thing to ask is: what is the primary aim of the trial?

## Randomisation, blinding and placebos

Some Phase II and nearly all Phase III trials are randomised. This mean that patients are randomly assigned to one arm of a trial or another – mostly this means either the new treatment versus a dummy drug in a placebo controlled trial, or new treatment versus standard of care. Randomisation is performed to reduce the risks of biasing the results of a trial – it is intended to avoid the temptation of investigators to give the new treatment to those patients they judge, consciously or unconsciously, to be most likely to benefit from it and therefore to skew the results.

Trials in which no randomisation takes place are often called 'open label' trials as everyone knows who is getting what and there is no control group. These trials are more subject to bias but still provide evidence for the effectiveness of a drug.

Blinded trials are those in which randomisation takes place but not all the parties involved know who is getting the new treatment and who isn't. In a single-blinded trial it is the patients who are unaware of whether they are being treated with the new treatment or the comparison (placebo or standard of care). The reason for doing this is that the patient's state of mind can play a part in the outcome and can therefore add bias to the results. For example patients who feel that they're on a new 'miracle' treatment may actually do better than they would otherwise – this is the placebo effect in action. In a double-blind trial neither the doctors nor the patients know who is getting the treatment – in this case it is to avoid the bias which may be introduced by doctors who interpret results more positively because they want the treatment to succeed or they believe in the 'miracle' drug too. These biases are not necessarily conscious or deliberate, but they do exist and therefore trying to factor them out means that the results are considered to be more objective. There are even triple-blinded trials, in which the statisticians who analyse the data from the different treatment arms do not know which group received the new treatment and which group didn't, in addition to the double-blinding of the doctors and patients on the trial.

A placebo drug is one that is designed to look and feel just like the drug being tested. Though often described as a 'sugar pill', a placebo drug can take many forms. It can be a liquid, capsule, injection and so on. In all cases where a placebo is used steps are taken so that the real drug and the placebo look exactly alike. The placebo effect describes the action of these dummy drugs – which can actually have positive physical effects on patients. Stress, fear, despair etc all have physical effects which can be reduced if a person's state of mind changes, and a placebo drug can do that. In a clinical trial it is important to separate the real effects of a treatment compared to the placebo effect, which is why the placebo drug is supposed to be indistinguishable from the real one.

In general the randomised, controlled, double-blinded Phase III trial is considered to have the least risk of bias and the results are given extra weight compared to unblinded or non-randomised trials. The majority of large Phase III trials are designed in this way in order to provide the strongest level of evidence before a treatment becomes standard of care. However, even such trials may be subject to bias or variance, so often a new treatment will undergo multiple Phase III trials and the data from them can then be looked at as a group in what is known as a meta-analysis.

## Conclusion

This chapter has outlined some of the most important information regarding the design and structure of clinical trials. It has highlighted the key questions that you need to ask if you are referred to a clinical trial, or if you are looking for a trial yourself. The next article in this series will examine in some detail the process of searching for a trial and some of the practical issues involved in joining a suitable trial.

## Summary

- Not all clinical trials are testing new treatments – some are about learning more about diseases, patient concerns, psychological interventions and so on

- It is always important to understand what the key outcomes of a treatment-related clinical trial are – is it looking at a curative treatment, is it aimed at reducing side effects or something else?
- Trials are often classed by Phase – though not all trials do this
- Phase 0 – These are testing very low doses of a new drug in a small number of patients to check for safety – not looking for any evidence of effect
- Phase 1 – Trials looking for the right dose to use in a later trial that looks for effectiveness. Main focus is on toxicity, secondary focus on therapeutic effect
- Phase 2 – These are the first trials which look for evidence of a therapeutic effect. They may or may not have a comparison group of patients to compare against
- Phase 3 – These are normally large randomised controlled trials. Some patients will get the new treatment and some will get a dummy drug (placebo) or the standard treatment. Often the final phase before a new treatment is licensed
- Phase 4 – This phase is about collecting additional data after a treatment has been licensed
- Randomisation – The process of randomly selecting patients to get the new treatment or

a placebo or standard of care. Designed to reduce the risk of biasing results

- Blinding – This is where the doctors and/or patients do not know which patients are receiving the new treatment and which the placebo or standard of care
- Placebo – A dummy drug that looks just like the real drug being tested

# Accessing Clinical Trials

## Introduction

In the previous chapter we looked at the design of clinical trials – what it is they seek to do, how they are classified by phase and how they are randomised or blinded. In this chapter we will be exploring the practical issues involved in joining a clinical trial – from how to find an appropriate trial to some of the difficulties in participation and finally looking at some of the alternative routes open to patients who cannot join trials.

Before looking at these issues in more detail, there is one question that is worth addressing immediately – if there are promising treatments available, why can't doctors prescribe them on an ad hoc basis? Why is a trial necessary? The answer is that it very much depends on the treatment being proposed.

Some drugs which are being tested at the moment in cancer treatments are actually well-known and well-characterised non-cancer drugs. The re-use of these drugs in cancer treatment is called 'drug repurposing' and includes many common drugs including aspirin, metformin and statins. Other such drugs include lesser known but still common drugs such as the anti-parasitic drug mebendazole, the anti-alcohol abuse drug disulfiram and the antibiotic clarithromycin (this topic is covered in more detail in the chapter on drug repurposing). Although these are well known drugs that are easily available on the NHS and, in some cases even available over the counter and without prescription, they are not licensed for cancer treatment. Any doctor who wants to prescribe these drugs as part of a cancer treatment is able to do so, but the drugs are being used 'off-label', which is problematic for some doctors. Many doctors prefer not to use drugs off-label and will wait for the conclusion of clinical trials and, hopefully, subsequent licensing of these drugs so that the use of them is firmly 'on-label' usage.

Of course many trials are using entirely new drugs which have not been licensed for any disease yet and which are not available to prescribe to patients. The drug companies producing these new drugs make them available for use in the controlled conditions of clinical trials. Even if a doctor wanted to use these drugs for a patient they are not able to access them. However, as we shall discuss in a later section, there are some limited circumstances in which some drugs which are authorised for clinical trial use can be made available to patients.

Finally, there are also cases of trials which are using existing cancer drugs, which are licensed for one form of the disease, being tried in a different cancer type. Generally these are well-known cancer drugs and they are often available to oncologists to prescribe 'off-label' in other cancer types outside of a clinical trial. Again, doctors are able to do this, although the practice is down to the discretion of the oncologist and subject to review from the multi-disciplinary team meeting which oversees cancer treatments in most centres.

The bottom line is that there are numerous cases where the use of a treatment that is being explored in a clinical trial may be accessed by patients outside of a trial. However, for many oncologists the clinical trial is the preferred mechanism for accessing new treatment options.

## Eligibility criteria

At heart a clinical trial is an experiment designed to answer one or more very specific questions. However, there is always a challenge to prove that the specific treatment or intervention really is causing the effects that are seen in the trial – how can we be sure that the observed effects aren't due to chance or the random variation in patients? This is particularly the case in Phase II and Phase III trials with multiple arms and a control group. Obviously one of the ways to control for these random variations in patient populations is to try and recruit patients where you can limit as much as possible those variations. By the same token, we also want the results of a trial to be generalizable to the real world, no matter how messy and variable it is. This is one of the key tensions in clinical trial design – trying to find the right balance that can show a measureable effect but not being so picky about patients that you cannot recruit enough of them or that they are totally unrepresentative of the real disease population.

One of the key features of each trial is the number of patients that it aims to recruit. This is called the sample size, with the idea being that the patients are a sample of the total population who will be eligible for the treatment being tested should it be successful. Sometimes the total population will be very wide – all patients with solid tumours, for example – and sometimes the total population will be very narrow – stage IV non-small cell lung cancer patients with a given genetic mutation in their tumours. However, the need to be able to detect the effect of the drug may mean that the trial designers want to try and limit real-world patient variability by adding additional constraints so that they can be more certain that the effect is down to the treatment and not a random by-product of something else. In real terms of course this means that each trial has a set of criteria to decide whether a given person matches the required profile for the sample.

Eligibility criteria describe those conditions that a patient must meet to be considered for the trial and is expressed in both positive and negative terms as *inclusion* and *exclusion* criteria. Common examples of inclusion criteria include age, gender, specific disease type (and, in the case of cancer, sub-type), current life-expectancy, a specific performance status (a measure of fitness) and so on. For exclusion criteria some common examples include certain previous treatments, specific current medication, poor blood markers, pregnancy or breastfeeding etc.

There are of course some serious downsides to selectivity, both for the patient and for medicine as a whole. For the patient the eligibility criteria are a significant hurdle which can often mean that access to an otherwise ideal clinical trial is not an option. In the cases of life-threatening diseases such as cancer, this denial of access can be a real blow and may leave a patient with no other obvious options to turn to. However, there may be some opportunity to access drugs off-trial, which we shall explore later.

The cost to society of having eligibility criteria that are too narrow can also be high. While restricting patient eligibility may mean that a trial can detect a positive effect of a treatment with relatively few patients in the sample, the very fact that the patients are so alike may mean that the results do not generalise to the rest of the population that the treatment is intended for. This means that treatments which appear to be incredibly promising, based on the results of these trials, actually do very little in the broader population or in larger trials. One response to this process has been a move towards a type of trial called a 'pragmatic clinical trial', to contrast with the 'explanatory clinical trial' which is the traditional model. A pragmatic trial has very little filtering of patients in an effort to match the real world, but the downside is that it becomes more difficult to detect small improvements in outcomes during the trial.

## Searching for clinical trials

In general patients (or their relatives or friends) do not go searching out clinical trials unless there is a problem. While some patients may be enrolled on clinical trials by their oncologist during first-line treatment – this can happen with some large Phase III trials which are testing a new protocol against the 'standard of care' – mostly clinical trials are viewed as an option when standard treatments fail. This can be after first or second-line treatment. Usually it is a process that is initiated by the oncology team rather than the patient. However, in some cases the process is initiated by the patient who wants to be proactive when he or she sees that a treatment is not working. In any case we will assume for this chapter that it is the patient who is actively looking for trial options.

If a patient is being treated in a large cancer centre then it is likely that a number of clinical trials are being carried out on-site, some of them may even involve their oncologist. In many of the larger centres there is usually a doctor who heads a clinical trials team. This team is often the first port of call when an oncologist wishes to look for a clinical trial for a patient. If your own oncologist has not already done so, then it is advisable to seek a consultation with this team as part of your search process. Obviously the pool of trials in any given centre, even a very large centre, is likely to be limited, but the clinical trials team will also be aware of trials in other centres, including some which can be accessed by their own patients.

Even with a clinical trials team on hand, it makes sense for a patient to search as widely as possible so that they are aware of the full range of possibilities which are being investigated for their own disease. This means looking at the full landscape of trials across the world, not limiting the search to your own locality or even country. Luckily there are a number of very good clinical trial registries or databases which can easily be accessed. We will look at each very briefly before looking at the search strategies which can be used to maximise the benefit of the available data.

### Clinicaltrials.gov

Clinicaltrials.gov is a global database and registry of clinical trial information from across the world. A service of the US National Institutes of Health (NIH), the database can be accessed by clinicians and members of the public from across the world. It features a simple query interface much like a search engine (like a specialised Google for clinical trials), but an advanced query screen – with many more options – is also available via the following URL: https://clinicaltrials.gov/ct2/search/advanced.

Trials can be searched by disease, location, trial status (e.g. currently recruiting patients), phase, age group and even who is funding the trial. It is thus possible to very quickly home in on trials that may be of interest to you. What is more, it is easy to refine a search so that you can add or remove search terms to increase or decrease the number of 'hits'.

For each 'hit' returned from a search there is a corresponding set of pages which give very detailed information about that trial. The basic header information includes the trial title, who the sponsor is (along with any collaborating organisations), a unique NCT identifier (e.g. NCT02022358) and the dates when the trial information was first added to the database and when it was last updated. More importantly there is information about the purpose of the trial, often with some information about the rationale behind it, as well as details of the specific disease, intervention (treatment) and the phase. Other information included will cover the primary and secondary outcome measures, the size of the trial in terms of patient numbers to be recruited and estimates of completion dates. There is also usually detailed information of the intervention being tested – and for multi-arm trials there will be details of the treatments in each arm. This information will often include timing and doses of drugs and some information of the protocol to be used.

Also of key importance for patients considering a trial is information on eligibility inclusion and exclusion criteria, as discussed previously. Finally there is often detailed information on contacts and locations. This will list not just the places where patients will be treated but, more important when searching for a trial, the names and, sometimes, the contact details of the key investigators. This is absolutely essential information for a patient seriously considering a trial – often a simple email is enough to initiate a conversation which can tell a patient whether the trial is worth following up or not.

Finally, some investigators also include links to relevant papers or documents which give more information on the rationale for the trial. This might be pre-clinical data or data from an earlier phase trial, or perhaps data from a similar trial in another type of cancer.

It is also worth noting that for some trials which have been completed the results are also included – sometimes on the results tab of the page, or sometimes as a link to a paper published in a peer-reviewed journal. These results can help identify whether the treatment being tested was successful or not. Unfortunately there are far too few results published in such accessible forms. However, for a completed study without results it is certainly advisable to email the contacts listed on the page to ask about the results – it may be that they have been published or delivered at a conference and nobody has updated the database.

Finally, for the tech savvy readers, it is worth noting that searches can be turned into a data feed using RSS so that updates and changes can be tracked automatically from within a web browser or RSS-compliant software.

## UK Clinical Trials Gateway

While clinicaltrials.gov is a service provided for by the US National Institutes of Health, there is also a UK equivalent which is provided for by the National Health Service via the National Institute of Health Research. The site can be accessed via the following URL: http://www.ukctg.nihr.ac.uk/. There are also apps which are provided for Android and iOS devices.

The basic search option on the home page allows for simple keyword searches – e.g. 'recurrent glioblastoma' or 'metastatic breast cancer'. Results are returned both in the form of a UK map with clickable locations and a listing by trial. The listing of trials is filtered by recruitment status: completed/recruiting/not recruiting/stopped. Each listed trial has an associated page with a similar level of information to the clinicaltrials.gov site – including eligibility, end-points, intervention details and contact information. Much of this information is sourced from the US site, and most of the trials have an NCT identifier and in fact there are hyperlinks on the UK site directly to clinicaltrials.gov.

In addition to the basic search, there is an advanced search option that allows searching by recruitment status, location, disease condition, intervention (for example surgery or the name of a specific drug) etc.

The information available from the UKCTG site is directly comparable to the information from clincialtrials.gov, though the trials listed are those that are in the UK. International trials with a UK arm are also included. Certainly navigating the results from the UKCTG site is easier, particularly in that you can see at a glance where trials are located in the UK. However, for a more global view of the trials landscape the US site is preferable.

### NCI Clinical Trials Search
Both of the registries mentioned above cover all medical conditions, not just cancer. The US National Cancer Institute (NCI) also hosts a search engine for clinical trials in cancer only. This can be accessed via the URL: http://www.cancer.gov/clinicaltrials/search.

This search engine accesses the same basic data as the other two registries, but has some additional features which make it worth considering. The first is that it is optimised for searching very specific cancer diagnoses – not just by disease sub-type but also by disease staging. It uses drop downs to select from cancer type and then offers check-boxes for disease stage. Location allows selection by country and city – though the interface defaults to US states and cities. It is a very clean interface and gets results very quickly. The only quirk to point out is that there is a sponsor field which defaults to *NIH*, change this to *All* to get the widest range of results.

It has some other nice touches, such as the ability to select from a wide selection of trial types (e.g. treatment, prevention, supportive care etc.), and an interface to easily pick from a database of drugs and so on. While the information returned largely matches the information from the other registries, the NCI interface scores well on user friendliness.

International Clinical Trials Registry Platform

The World Health Organisation also hosts an international registry of clinical trials – with a broader set of data to choose from than clinicaltrials.gov and the UKCTG. The range includes the US, EU, Australia/ New Zealand, China, Japan and more. The URL to access the database is: http://apps.who.int/trialsearch/.

The basic search option includes the support of wild-cards and logical operators in searches. For example 'breast cancer AND celecoxib' will search for all breast cancer trials which include the drug celecoxib. Other logical operators include OR and NOT. The asterisk is the wild-card character, so 'liv*' will search for 'liver' and 'Liverpool'.

Results returned cannot be filtered and the basic search will return trials in all countries and with all recruitment stages. The advanced search page gives greater control over searching and can specify countries, recruitment status, sponsors and so on, in addition to the logical operators in the key words.

The core information (phase, treatment type, country etc) is included in all listed clinical trials, usually with links back to local registries which have more information. The format is less user-friendly than the sites mentioned previously, but the fact remains that the sheer spread of information cannot be matched elsewhere.

## EU Clinical Trials Register

The final international registry to cover briefly is the one supplied by the European Union and hosted by the European Medicines Agency. The URL is: https://www.clinicaltrialsregister.eu.

In terms of user interface this is most familiar to the WHO site, as is the output. In fact the information from this registry is included in the WHO site – therefore use of this site is useful only in that it simplifies searching for European trials as they can be searched in one go. Otherwise the WHO site is preferable.

## Other Registries

So far all the registries listed have been provided by national or international health agencies, but there are also other sources of information which are of some considerable value. Not all clinical trials are included in the registries mentioned previously – there are also many small trials which are taking place in hospitals and clinics which are not registered centrally. Very often these are early phase trials with new agents and typically only involve one or two centres; however, they are certainly worth considering when options are limited.

The best place to find information on these trials is with the companies which sponsor them. A number of pharmaceutical companies run their own clinical trial registries and provide websites which list the details. It is not simply large pharma companies which do this, there are a number of medium and small companies which also run websites that provide useful trial information. It is beyond the scope of this document to list these private registries, however, a generic approach to finding this information would be more useful.

The starting point is generally an interest in a specific drug – possibly as a result of an article in a newspaper, science website or medical journal (or from a Pubmed search). Once you have the name of the drug it is not difficult to find out which company is developing it. From there it's normally enough to do a web search on the name of the company and the phrase 'clinical trials' or 'clinical trials registry'.

As an example let's take the new drug vismodegib, which is an example of a class of drugs called Hedgehog pathway inhibitors. A quick search brings up the Wikipedia page which lists the company Genentech as the developer of the drug. A second search of 'genentech clinical trials' eventually takes us to the web site for Genentech's trials: http://www.genentechclinicaltrials.com/.

## Compassionate Use

As has been mentioned previously, every clinical trial has a set of inclusion and exclusion criteria. Unfortunately this often means that patients find they cannot be admitted to a trial that is investigating the use of a drug or other treatment for their specific disease. However, this need not be the end of the line as far as that treatment is concerned, and there is a mechanism in place that can, in certain circumstances, mean that a patient can have access to the drug outside of the trial. This is through a mechanism called a 'compassionate use' programme.

Many pharmaceutical companies developing cancer drugs actually run compassionate use programmes, in which they supply the newest drugs which they are trialling to patients who cannot otherwise access them. As would be expected there are very strict conditions associated with these programmes. First and most obvious is that a patient should be suffering from a serious and life-threatening condition. Second, the patient must have been through all standard treatments and have no other viable treatment options open to him or her. This also means that there are no open clinical trials that the patient can join. Finally, the request for compassionate use must come from the patient's treating physician – not the patient, family member or advocate.

These are actually fairly stringent conditions. It means that a patient cannot attempt to gain compassionate use access without first persuading his or her oncologist that it is a good idea. There may be considerable administrative work involved in gaining such access, and many oncologists do not have experience of these programmes. There is also a certain hesitation from some doctors to try new options outside of a trial. In any case, regardless of the oncologist's feelings on the matter, a person has every right to push for treatment options that may help their condition. Although it may be difficult to argue a case with an oncologist, it may become necessary when exploring this type of programme.

It may be worth contacting the pharmaceutical company's compassionate use programme directly in the first instance. Again this is a way of speeding up a process that might otherwise drag on. An initial contact will clarify many questions and may indicate whether it would be worth exploring the option via the treating oncologist or not.

The strict conditions also mean that a patient cannot attempt to access a drug through compassionate use if there is another trial open that he or she could join. This condition applies even if the open trial does not appear to be as positive or promising as the drug available on the compassionate use programme.

Assuming that the conditions are met, and the application is made via the treating oncologist, access may only be granted in the cases where the drug company has sufficient supplies of the drug (which is not always the case with new drugs that are not yet being manufactured). The company will also need to be satisfied that the clinic or hospital treating the patient has specifically agreed the compassionate use for that patient (i.e. that the doctor making the application on behalf of the patient has approval from an ethics committee or other relevant body at the hospital).

## Early Access to Medicines Scheme

While compassionate access programmes are run by the drugs companies, there is also a new scheme in the UK which has recently been introduced by the Medicines and Healthcare Products Regulatory Agency (MHRA). This scheme is intended to provide early access to new medicines for patients with life-threatening or seriously debilitating conditions for which there are clear unmet medical needs. The aim is to give these patients access to medicines which have not been fully licensed but which have been designated as promising innovative medicines (PIMs). The scheme is intended to fast track the most promising new drugs to the areas of greatest medical needs.

How this new scheme develops in the future will be of great interest to cancer patients, but for now it is too early to say whether this will succeed or not.

## Summary

- Clinical trials try to balance the need to reduce patient variability with the need to have a representative sample of patients
- All trials have eligibility criteria – both inclusion and exclusion criteria are used to select the sample of patients recruited onto the trial
- Clinical trial registries are online databases that allow people to search for suitable trials. Typical search criteria include disease type, phase of trial, trial recruitment status and physical location
- Search results will give detailed information on the trial, including eligibility criteria, details of the treatment and often the contact details of the primary investigators running the trial

- In addition to the public registries, such as clinicaltrials.gov or the UK clinical trials gateway, there are also registries published by some of the companies developing new drugs and treatments
- Patients who do not meet eligibility criteria might still qualify to receive the drug off-trial on a compassionate use basis

# How to Assess a Medical Paper – Preclinical Data

## Introduction

This chapter is aimed at the scientifically literate reader who isn't a medic or a biochemist. It's aimed at those patients and families who are undertaking to read the research directly in the hope of finding something useful for their own situation. It will provide pointers to the best places to go to find suitable scientific papers as well as a picture of the typical architecture of a medical paper. More importantly it will provide advice on how to interpret the content of those papers – in other words how to make sense of some of that vast and growing literature on cancer.

In addition to assuming that the reader is not an expert in medicine or biochemistry, this chapter assumes that the reader is primarily interested in assessing the evidence for or against various treatment options rather than being interested in an academic understanding of cancer. Furthermore, many of the examples assume that the reader is looking for evidence of effect from different drugs, foods, vitamins, minerals and dietary supplements –

experience has shown that many cancer patients and their carers are looking for precisely this sort of information in the cancer literature.

Be prepared for a shock when you first start reading the peer-reviewed medical literature on cancer. When you first dip your toe in the waters you will be struck by the vast number of papers that show how cancer cells are wiped out by this, that or other treatment. Whether it be plant polyphenols like curcumin or quercetin, vitamins like C or D3, or medicinal mushrooms like Ganoderma Lucidum or... The list is endless, and so are the papers. There are hundreds of thousands of them in fact, with a never ending supply of new publications arriving every day. So why is it that cancer is still a problem? Why is it that curcumin or quercetin or EGCG or any of the other natural agents and food supplements haven't cured cancer? If we believe all of these papers, it should have been cured by now – the results are that clear. The answer is complex, and it isn't down to Big Pharma having killed the research or drowned the scientists or to any other favourite conspiracy theory (see the chapter on Cancer and the Media for more on conspiracy theories and cancer).

This chapter is specifically looking at pre-clinical data – that is data from different types of experiments and studies performed *before* you get to running tests of a drug or treatment in humans. This normally means laboratory experiments of various kinds.

## What Is A Medical Paper?

This may seem like an odd starting place, but it is important to be clear about what we mean by a paper on cancer. The fact is that there are many documents published which may appear to be academic papers on various aspects of medicine, particularly relating to cancer. A quick search on Google or Bing is likely to bring up thousands of hits which appear to fit the bill: they are filled with technical jargon, scientific diagrams and are structured to look like real academic papers. However it is always important to verify that the content is actually from a *peer-reviewed journal*. What does peer-review mean? It is the process by which a scientific journal provides a form of quality check on an article before it is published. Before being accepted for publication an article is sent to a number of experienced scientists and experts so that they can review the content to ensure that it is accurate, that it makes sense and that it conforms to the standards expected in the field. While it does not mean that every article that goes through peer review is error free, it does at least pass through a process in which the authors can be asked to clarify, amend or provide additional evidence for a claim they are making. It is this peer review process which makes scientific publishing different to most other forms of publication.

However, as one would expect there are costs involved in the process of publishing scientific journals. Therefore it is usual practice for scientists to have to defer some of these costs by paying an article processing fee. These fees vary depending on the journal but they can be considerable – often exceeding £1500 per article. This income stream has attracted the attentions of numerous scammers who create fake peer-reviewed journals with the intention of conning researchers into handing over these processing fees. Some of these journals are very sophisticated in that they are backed up by impressive looking websites, prestigious office addresses, distinguished names on their review boards and lists of realistic looking papers. These journals are known as 'predatory journals' and they are increasing in both number and sophistication. What is worse is that some unscrupulous people peddling fake cancer cures or therapies, with dubious levels of evidence are using these journals to publish papers which promote the products or therapies they are selling.

For this reason it is essential that you access medical papers from reputable sources, starting with PubMed (http://www.ncbi.nlm.nih.gov/pubmed), which is the world's number one search engine and online database for biomedical literature. In contrast to Google Scholar, for example, the papers listed in a PubMed search are from established peer-reviewed journals. What is more, many of these can be downloaded or accessed directly via PubMed or links to the original journal.

## Structure of a Medical Paper

While there are obvious variations in style and content, on the whole most medical papers follow a set pattern in terms of structure. This is sometimes called the IMRAD format – Introduction, Methods, Results and Discussion. The Introduction is designed to set the scene for the paper – it outlines the reason for the clinical trial or problem the paper is discussing. The Method section deals with the nuts and bolts of how the experiments were performed, or it outlines the protocol in a clinical trial. The Results section is where the data is presented. Discussion is what it says – a discussion of the results and how they should be interpreted. Often the Discussion section will also discuss the limitations of a trial or series of experiments, as well as attempting to outline the significance of the results in a broader context.

Additionally, each paper includes an Abstract and a set of References. The Abstract is probably the key thing to look at when searching through lots of academic papers. It is a succinct summary of the paper – with a précis of the problem, outline of key experiments, the headline results and a short conclusion. It's the essence of the paper distilled into one or two paragraphs. The References lists all the other academic papers and sources that the authors of the paper have cited – it means that readers can track back to related information, pre-existing data or other scientists publishing on the same topic.

For the non-expert reader some of these sections of a paper are more interesting than others. Typically the Abstract, Introduction, Results and Discussion are where you will gain most value and have most chance of understanding. The Method section tends to be the most technical, though it often contains key information on drug dosages, clinical trial protocols and so on.

Having outlined what an academic paper looks like we can now assess the content of different types of study of interest to cancer patients and carers.

## What is pre-clinical research for?
Before looking at the two most common forms of pre-clinical study, *in vitro* and *in vivo*, we ought to briefly touch on some of the main reasons for carrying out such research. Firstly it should be

obvious that there is much that we don't understand about cancer biology. While our understanding of molecular biology has expanded rapidly in the last couple of decades there is still much that is still a mystery to scientists. One mechanism to get a handle on the complexity of a living system is to try and create simple experiments in controlled conditions – and one of the simplest is to use cells growing in petri dishes. Here the conditions can be controlled and changes in cells observed using advanced technology. It's a powerful tool to understand what is going on *inside* individual cells. For example it's a good way to understand how given chemicals act on cells – do the cells survive, do they stop multiplying, do they continue to absorb nutrients etc. For scientists looking at the effects of drugs they can use this kind of study to see how the cells respond to different concentrations of the drug. In other cases scientists are not looking at the effect of drugs but are trying to work out the very detailed workings of different kinds of cells, for example trying to understand all of the steps involved in cells communicating with each other in response to changes in environmental conditions.

But of course cells grown in cultures are a long way from cells in living beings. Therefore, there is also a lot of research performed in animals. Much of this is a progression from experiments performed in cell cultures. If we stay with the example of testing drugs, it is normally the case that once researchers have established in cell cultures that a treatment has the specific effect they are looking for they'll test the drug in animals to see if they can reproduce it. Sometimes it happens the other way too – they will have evidence from animal experiments that a drug works, but will resort to a simplified cell culture system to work out exactly *how* it is doing it.

Ultimately for the type of research that is focused on cancer treatments, the experiments in cell cultures and in animals are necessary steps along the way to using the treatment in people. It is important to keep in mind the rationale for this type of research when looking at the results in papers.

## In Vitro Studies

In vitro studies make up a large part of the published literature on cancer. Vitro is Latin for glass, so literally in this context in vitro studies expose cancer cells in glass tubes or dishes to different substances – from drugs to vitamins, minerals, herbs etc – to see what happens. The first thing to note is that in the vast majority of papers that are published on cancer and substance X (where X is whatever is being tested) the results tend to show that X will kill cancer cells. Frequently it is found that cancer cells in test tubes are killed by all sorts of common (and not so common) substances – plant extracts, yeasts, mushrooms, herbs, minerals, fruits, berries, vegetables and more.

This may seem very encouraging at first. It's great. Who would not be happy to find that a common substance like curcumin or vitamin C can kill cancer cells? Even better if you can find that it kills the particular type of cancer you're interested in. The bone cancer osteosarcoma, for example, is susceptible to curcumin, quercetin, EGCG, genistein, sulforaphane and more. It's not just plant extracts. There are plenty of papers showing that commonly used non-cancer drugs, such as celecoxib, are also potent anti-osteosarcoma drugs. Osteosarcoma isn't unique here, for every type of cancer there are papers that show dozens of different substances have potent activity in the test tube.

However, there are some key things that have to be kept in mind when reading these papers. First and most obvious is that a test tube is not the same as a live body. It's not even the same as a live tumour come to that. A live tumour contains lots of different types of cells, it's surrounded by a whole supporting eco-system of cells (commonly called the tumour microenvironment or stroma), and it interacts with an immune system and is supplied with blood and nutrients. Most of these are not present during in vitro studies. What you have is pretty much a thin film of cancer cells sitting on a growth medium – which is a long way from cancer cells out in the wild.

Secondly, these carefully nurtured cancer cells are then exposed to a very closely monitored dose of the candidate substance or drug. Not only is the dose carefully calculated, the length of this exposure is carefully controlled too. Very often the substance being tested is used at such high doses and for sustained periods that it is physiologically impossible to achieve (at least without killing the human or animal patient).

Yet another issue that is relevant is the specific form of substance X that is being tested. In the majority of cases the experiments use a purified form of the substance, often dissolved in solvent or processed in some way. Again this is a problem if you are looking for foods or nutritional supplements because of the obvious reason that you or I will have to swallow and metabolise the substance. This means that what passes out of the gut into the bloodstream is not the same substance as that being tested in the lab. For example, most in vitro studies of the anti-cancer effect of curcumin use pure curcumin rather than the metabolites that are produced as a result of our digestive processes.

Finally, attention also has to be paid to the particular cell lines being used in these in vitro studies. It isn't enough to say that a study has used breast (or prostate or osteosarcoma or whatever) cells – you need to know the exact sub-type of the disease. And even with the right sub-type, you need to know what characteristics these cells express – what is the p53 status? Is it hormone responsive? Does it express COX-2 or other inflammatory markers? Does it have high or low metastatic potential? All of these are important questions, and of course you need to know some of those answers for your own disease. Why? Because it's not uncommon to find that an in vitro study is performed against a panel of different cells lines and that there are good results for some, and poor results for others, even though all of the cell lines are breast or prostate or other type of cancer. Or, just as common, two different sets of experiments exist, performed by different teams using the same cell lines and they'll report opposite conclusions.

Unfortunately what this means is that the startling results in the test tube almost never translate to our bodies. The in vitro study tests an artificial system of cancer cells with impossibly high levels of a pure substance that wouldn't pass through our digestive systems no matter how much of it we swallowed. To all intents and purposes this means that you have to take these test tube studies with a huge pinch of salt. In the test tube substance X kills cancer, but that really doesn't mean much in the real world. At most it gives you reasons to carry on looking at substance X in more detail. Very often this is *precisely* the result that the researchers were looking for. Remember that the rationale for much of this work is to take it on to the next stage of research.

You may well ask, if this is the case then why are so *many* in vitro studies being performed? What is the point? It's a good question.

Firstly, and most obviously, in vitro studies are relatively easy to perform. Compared to doing animal or human studies in vitro studies are easy. There are no ethics committees to convince, there's no hassle of dealing with animals (and thanks to the activities of 'animal liberationists' there are no major security worries either) and the results can come out quickly. For a beginning researcher, or a department looking at its publication record (and probably funding applications), this is a simple way of getting published. This isn't being cynical, scientists are people too and they've got other pressures to worry about as well as trying to make progress against cancer. Getting a few good papers published adds weight to a PhD thesis and it looks good on a departmental publication record. On the plus side it can also spark off other interesting ideas for new research. It's also worth pointing out that there are many in the animal rights lobby who are actively working to increase the amount of in vitro work going on because it saves the lives of laboratory animals. The focus on saving animal lives obscures the fact that many of the results of in vitro experiments are of academic interest only and don't translate well to animals or humans.

However, most importantly in vitro research can provide details of how things work, giving us more data and a greater level of understanding of the processes that go on at a very detailed level. When a relatively new substance, a rare plant extract for example or some fancy new molecule is discovered, then the research has got to start somewhere. This is a quick way of knowing whether it's worth exploring in any more depth or not. When you want to elucidate how particular molecular pathways interact, or you want to understand which proteins are produced by cells in specific circumstances – in other words you are interested in detailed biochemical analyses – then in vitro work is ideal. But if your aim is to see if substance X kills cancer Y at dose Z then in vitro studies are so far removed from what happens inside people that the results are barely relevant.

There are those who are working hard at addressing some of the pit-falls that I've outlined previously. For example there are groups of researchers working on producing tumour spheroids under glass – in other words they want to produce 3-dimensional tumours in vitro, making them more like the real thing. There are also experiments where the metabolites of curcumin or other substances are used and not just the pure raw material. And of course there are those in vitro studies where the researchers go out of their way to only use physiologically achievable doses. This is all to the good, but as a reader of that research you have to be on the look-out for these. Another strand of activity is in silico studies, where researchers use sophisticated software to test how different molecules connect with each other – again useful as a first step but a million miles from the insides of a living, breathing person.

## In Vivo Studies

The next step up from in vitro are in vivo studies – in other words studies that take place in living tissue rather than in a petri dish. For the most part these studies use rats and mice, though sometimes you'll find other animals being used. Again we will focus on cancer research of the sort that looks at what effect a given substance has on cancer rather than on research trying to understand how cancer develops and spreads, for example.

The good news is that if you are a rat or a mouse there has never been a better time to have cancer. Again and again we see fantastic results in rodents. Cancers of many different sorts are slowed, stopped, destroyed. It is impossible not to feel excited by some of these results, and they are truly remarkable. Unfortunately however, these fantastic results on lab rats do not translate as well to humans. Why is that? We saw that test tube studies have all kinds of issues – surely these problems disappear once you move from glass dishes to living beings?

Some of the disadvantages of the test tube approach are easily solved in rats, mice and other animals. No longer do you have just a flat layer of cancer cells to bathe in your anti-cancer agent. Instead you have three-dimensional tumours embedded in tissue, with a blood supply and tumour microenvironment. And, interestingly enough, we find that some agents that have fantastic results in the test tube are all of a sudden not so powerful against tumours in animals. Instead the same agents have lower efficacy and in some cases seem to have lost all trace of anti-cancer effect. Why? Because the high dosing and carefully controlled test tube conditions cannot be transferred to a living being. Doses that killed tumour cells under glass can also be toxic to living animals. In some cases you find that there is what is termed a biphasic response – at the low dose that can be achieved in animals the agent turns out to be *pro-cancerous*, and at the higher dose it does kill the tumours but also kills the animals or makes them seriously sick. Not good.

However, there are also cases when the results in animals are good. Tumours that are growing fast are slowed down substantially, or else they stop growing completely or even regress and disappear. Let's be clear, each of these responses is significant. Having an agent that slows growth is important, some cancers are highly aggressive so slowing them down is important. Having a tumour stop growing (which is normally what doctors would class as stable disease), is a major achievement. And having tumours shrink and eventually die is precisely what we want. So, while these positive responses are not as common as those great results you see in test tube studies, they are striking nevertheless and should give us grounds for optimism. It's not hard to find studies that show that curcumin, quercetin, sodium bicarbonate, ascorbic acid (vitamin C) and plenty of other agents can deliver positive results in rats.

Onwards to human trials and similar positive results – right? Unfortunately not. History is littered with stellar pre-clinical results that have not translated well into clinical practice. Anti-angiogenic therapies, to take one well-known example, work by stopping tumours sprouting the blood supply they need to survive. In mice and rats it often works, in humans...well, it's never worked the way the rat models suggest it should. Why? As with the in vitro results, we need to dig below the surface to uncover the major problems with in vivo results.

The first thing to note is that a mouse is a mouse, a rat is a rat and a human is something else altogether. Mice and rats don't get human cancers. A mouse will get murine cancer, in the same way that dogs are prone to canine cancers and we are prone to human cancers. And, for the purposes of experimentation you can't afford to wait around for your mouse to develop cancer by chance (called *spontaneous* cancers in the jargon). In practice this means chemically inducing cancer or the use of genetically engineered mice.

Genetically engineered mice are specially bred to spontaneously develop murine cancers – in other words their DNA is changed so that they have a very high risk of developing cancer. This ensures a supply of mouse patients that can be used to explore how the disease develops or, more usefully, what works in stopping the mice getting sick in the first place. If your interest is in the process of metastasising, then you can watch how the tumours spontaneously develop in these mice, how they progress and then metastasise to other parts of the body. This is very useful in terms of understanding how these things happen, and there is an awful lot that we don't know even at very basic levels. However, these are mice cancers, not human. If you're testing a new treatment, translating from this type of mouse model to human disease is simply not reliable.

An alternative approach is to use what are called *xenograft* models. Here you take a mouse and inject a human cancer into it. This becomes the target of investigation and treatments are assessed against these human cancers and not mouse ones. But doing this is not straightforward for two simple reasons. First and most obvious is that the mouse immune system is fairly good at rejecting transplanted human cells, even cancer cells. So it's not easy to get human cancers to grow in a fully immune-competent mouse.

Secondly, and less obviously, the cells that are transplanted are not always fully representative of human cancers either. Again, as was pointed out previously, standard cell lines of the type that are supplied by cell libraries represent only one cell type. Tumours contain many different cells types, they are not just a blob of identical cancer cells – real tumours contain multiple populations of cancer cells, immune cells and other non-cancer cells. Cancer cells mutate and adapt, so cells that have been taken from a patient biopsy twenty or thirty years ago, and then kept under glass for generation after generation, will have changed in order to survive in the test tube environment. In many cases these lab-grown human cancer cells no longer even resemble the cancers that they started out from many years ago, simply because they have evolved to survive in test tube conditions.

One way round the first issue of immune rejection is to engineer various types of mice with malfunctioning immune systems – these are called *immunodeficient* mice. There are different flavours of such mice: the athymic mouse, SCID (severe combined immunodeficiency) and so on. These different flavours of mice have become the model of choice for much cancer (and other disease) research. The immunodeficient mouse enables scientists to plant human cancers into the mice and then let the tumours develop. Furthermore, this ease of transplanting tumours means that scientists can take any type of cancer and plant it somewhere in the mouse – very often it's the flank because tumours there are easy to see and measure using callipers. Treatments can be assessed, basic research into the underlying biology can take place and we can learn a lot in the process.

But of course we are not dealing with the real thing, by changing the immune system we have removed a key component of real animals and real people. And, as is becoming increasingly clear as the science advances, in real cancer, the immune system is more than just an innocent bystander. Real tumours work in concert with the local environment, recruiting some types of immune cells, subverting others or just sending out all kinds of chemical signals and messages. Taking out the immune system removes this essential interplay.

Some of these problems are in the process of being addressed. For example, there is an increasing use of *orthotopic* xenograft models, where, for example, breast cancers are implanted in the mammary pads of mice, or osteosarcoma cells implanted in bone etc. These at least have the merit of being implanted in the same kind of tissues that they would in a human. It's a step in the right direction, but we still have the issue that these are being implanted in immunodeficient mice. It is also generally the case that these orthotopic tumours do not necessarily grow in the same way in the mouse than they do in humans.

The next step in the process is the development of mouse tumours that more closely resemble human tumours. These mouse tumours will have been engineered to express similar pathways, and carry similar mutations to human cancers. They will be implanted into fully immunocompetent mice, and develop with the mouse immune system in play. There are already examples of such systems available, though in comparison to immunodeficient mice the cost is considerably higher, as is the skill required to care for them. However, the evidence from these 'syngeneic mouse models' should be more highly rated than the evidence from xenograft evidence in immune-deficient mice.

So far we have just focused on how closely mice with cancer match the human disease. But there are other things to look at when reading the results of experiments where mice have been treated with different agents. As before, let's focus on the kind of substances that we can buy over the counter in supplement form: curcumin, quercetin, modified citrus pectin etc. The key question to ask is: how was the substance delivered?

As patients or family, we are often looking for evidence that taking something like curcumin or resveratrol has powerful anticancer activity. We've looked at the test tube results and are impressed.

Now we look at the mice and rat experiments and the results look good. But are they?

In many animal experiments the substance being tested is not given orally. Very often the substance being tested is injected intravenously or intraperitoneally (injected into the body cavity), or sometimes intramuscularly or subcutaneously. Often the substance has been dissolved in a solvent called DMSO or some other chemical. From the point of view of the experimenter this makes sense – they can guarantee the dose and control how much gets into the mouse. For us, this is not much help. We won't be looking to inject, we want to take it in tablet or powder form.

There are cases, however, where the dose is oral. Normally this is described as by *gavage* – in other words it is inserted into the stomach via a tube. In some papers you'll see that the agent is mixed into the diet or the drink and the mouse isn't force fed. These are the experiments that are most interesting from our point of view. Good results here are normally worth taking note of. There are some things to be aware of, the most obvious being the translation of a mouse dose to a human dose, but there are standard formulae for doing that.

So, have we found our perfect experiment? If mice eating substance X at dose Y show good results against the type of cancer we are interested in, does that mean we should go ahead and start taking substance X too? Unfortunately we have to come back again to looking at what types of mice were used…

Even if the results are good, you still need to know whether the mice were immunodeficient or not. You need to know whether the tumours were orthotopic or not. If human cancers were used, what subtype and how closely do the mice models match the human disease? You need to know what else was going on as regards diet and so on.

The point of all this is not to say that looking at mice models of cancer is no good. It's just that there are so many caveats and so many discrepancies between what goes on in us and what goes on in mice and rats that we need to exercise caution. Time and again promising results in mice turn out to be failures in human trials. We, as patients or carers, need to exercise the same caution as the drug companies should when looking at results.

This also begs the question of how many wrong turns science has taken because of the difficulties of using mouse models. Who knows how many positive results have been missed because the mice were missing key components of the immune system? And how much time has been lost because fantastic results disappear when the immune system does come into play?

Finally, if you do find some great results in your search, then the obvious next place to look is at human trials. And that's where we'll look in the next chapter.

## Summary

- Medical research is most often published in peer-reviewed medical journals in the form of articles or papers that follow a common format
- Beware of fake papers and fake journals which pretend to be based on science but are deliberately designed to deceive readers – use the PubMed search engine to look for peer reviewed papers
- Medical research that is described as pre-clinical refers to studies carried out in test tubes, petri dishes and animals – it is necessary to carry out this type of research to further our understanding of biology and also to test for safety and effectiveness before a treatment can be tried in people

- In vitro research takes place in test tubes and petri dishes – this can provide useful data but it's hard to extrapolate results from this type of research to humans
- In vivo research uses animals such as mice and rats – this also provides useful clues to whether something works as a cancer treatment, but it is not directly transferable to humans
- Positive results from pre-clinical data, both in vitro and in vivo, can lead on to clinical research

# How to Assess a Medical Paper - Human Data

## Introduction

In the previous chapter we looked at how we can evaluate data from the academic literature on laboratory (both in vitro and in vivo) experiments – which we can loosely think of as supplying the information that eventually leads to data in humans. It is human data that we are ultimately interested in and in this chapter we are going to be specifically considering data that is used to assess whether a given treatment intervention works or not. Not all published data is of this type – there are many clinical studies which are not looking at treatment options and are instead focused on understanding the underlying biology of cancer, the use of specific markers to gauge the state of the disease process or perhaps looking at predictive markers which can be used clinically to plan treatments and many other topics not directly related to the effectiveness (often referred to as efficacy) of different treatments.

The majority of the academic papers we will be considering in this chapter are reporting results from clinical trials. However, this is not the only sort of human data that is available. Two other notable sources of non-trial data are *case reports* and *epidemiological* data.

## Non-trial Data

Case reports are just that – formal reports of individual cases, sometimes only a single case, sometimes a small series of cases together. These reports are normally published because they illustrate something out of the ordinary that the doctors who have written them up want to make other doctors aware of. It could be that the cases represent very unusual symptoms, rare side effects of a treatment or even a very rare combination of diseases in one patient. However there are also published case reports which cover unusual responses to treatments, the use of drugs 'off-label' or remarkable cases of remissions in cancer. A good case report is usually well-documented with details of the disease, the treatment, radiological results (CT scans or x-rays) and so on. Obviously because the reports are only covering individual cases there is a limit to the conclusions we can draw from them – we certainly can't conclude that because one patient had a sustained cancer remission while take mebendazole (an anti-parasitic drug available over the counter) that all patients, or even the majority of patients, will also achieve the same results. At best these case reports are useful data for forming a hypothesis which should later be explored in a clinical trial, at worst some case reports are uninformative anecdotes which do not warrant much consideration.

This is not to say that individual case reports or a small series of reports are of no value in medicine. In some cases published case reports have triggered subsequent investigations and clinical trials. They can be important starting points, particularly in rare diseases or cancers for which there are few effective treatments. Indeed in some instances case reports have been followed up with positive clinical trials leading to changes in clinical practices that have benefited patients directly – and this continues to be the case, especially in diseases, including some cancers, in which there are no currently effective treatments.

The other form of non-trial data comes from epidemiological studies, often also called retrospective studies, in which data from different population groups are examined to see if there are any useful patterns regarding cancer incidence, outcomes and other measures of interest. Good examples include studies which have found that diabetic patients with cancer taking the drug metformin have better survival than similar patients taking other anti-diabetic drugs [1]. There is also data that shows that colorectal cancer patients who had been taking aspirin for heart attack prevention for a number of years had better outcomes than patients who hadn't been taking aspirin [2]. As with the best of the case reports, this can be useful data that builds up a rationale for a clinical trial, particularly when put together with some of the in vitro and in vivo pre-clinical data discussed in the previous chapter. However, finding these patterns in data is tricky and there are multiple statistical methods for analysing it – which means that different conclusions can arise from very similar datasets depending on which techniques you use to analyse it. And, as with all epidemiological data, it's very difficult to take account of all the possible confounding variables (the numerous other factors that can influence those data patterns). For example, many diabetic patients on metformin take extra care with their diets, they may do more exercise, may take other medications and so on – you need to make sure that the diabetic patients not on metformin do the same, otherwise it could be the diet and exercise making the difference, not the metformin.

In some cases retrospective studies are performed in which historical patient records are examined to answer very specific questions regarding treatment outcomes. For example, there have been a number of studies which have looked at the rate of recurrence or relapse in cancer patients who were treated with surgery, but who had different pain-killers during the surgical procedures [3]. The patient records are split into different groups based on the type of pain-killer used, and then comparisons made between them to see if there is a pattern related to this difference in treatment. This type of retrospective study is also often performed as a way of confirming that a hypothesis is worth exploring in a future clinical trial.

The bottom line is that while human non-clinical trial data is useful, it should be treated with caution and it often carries far less weight in medical practice than data gathered from clinical trials. However, some non-trial data provides a solid starting point for subsequent clinical trials, particularly in illnesses lacking effective treatments.

## Clinical Trial Data

Before diving in to look at how to interpret data from clinical trials, it might be best to make a detour first to the chapters on clinical trial design if you have not already read them. Much of what follows will make reference to different types of trial design, so if in doubt please refer back to the relevant sections of those chapters. Note that this data is from prospective or interventional trials, in contrast to the observational or retrospective studies mentioned above. These are studies in which the investigators intervene – they apply a treatment in other words, rather than just observing data or viewing historical records.

Unfortunately, assessing the *value* of data from clinical trials is not a straightforward task and even experts can often disagree in their assessments of the same data. That said, it is helpful to at least consider a few of the main determinants that we need to include in an assessment.

The first point to consider is the trial phase. In general, data from randomised controlled trials is judged to be of greater value than data from non-randomised or non-controlled trials. Keep in mind that in Phase I trials – which tend to be very small in oncology – what we are looking at is primarily data on the safety and toxicity of the treatment being tested. Sometimes positive results are included to show that the drug is not only tolerable but shows signs of clinically useful activity, but these should be judged cautiously. Phase I trials are not randomised, not placebo controlled and are subject to all sorts of biases – and because the numbers are small it is hard to know whether a positive result is a lucky fluke or a sign of real clinical effect.

Phase II trial data tends to be taken more seriously as this is when clinicians are first looking to see evidence of efficacy. Sometimes you'll see trials designated as Phase IIA or IIB – in the first case there is more focus on dosing, in the second there is more emphasis on efficacy. This means that data from Phase IIB trials is more important when looking to see whether a treatment is effective or not. Some Phase II trials are fully randomised – which in oncology means that some patients are assigned to receive the new treatment and some assigned to receive the standard treatment – and some are also double-blinded, which means that the doctors treating the patients do not know which patient is getting the new treatment and which the old. This process of randomising and blinding is intended to minimise the influence of biases which can skew the results. But note that not all Phase II trials are randomised or blinded, some can be non-randomised and open label, which means that everyone knows which patients are getting the new treatment. This does mean that results of such trials are treated with more caution, especially if the number of patients being treated is relatively small.

However, this does not mean that the results from Phase II trials are not taken seriously or are viewed as not having sufficient sway to change clinical practice. In many rarer forms of cancer patient populations are small, the unmet needs are high and it is often not feasible to go beyond Phase II trials. It is simply not true that it needs large Phase III trials to get a drug licensed for use or for practice to change – more than 50% of drug licences in cancer are granted by the authorities on the basis of well-designed and well-run Phase II clinical trials. If you are looking for evidence of effect for a less common cancer then Phase II data, particularly from randomised controlled trials, is perfectly acceptable as an evidence base.

In general however, most weight is given to Phase III clinical trials, in which patient numbers are considerably higher than in Phase II trials – often going over 1000 patients in the more common cancers. These larger patient numbers mean that the trial is carried out by multiple teams in different institutions and in different countries – this is good because it reduces the risk of unconscious bias introduced by very motivated groups in single centre studies. Where smaller studies are normally run by clinical researchers, in these larger trials it is normally ordinary clinicians who are treating the patients. And, given the size of the trial, it is more likely that the patients match the general population of patients with the disease being investigated rather than the more carefully selected patients in the earlier phase trials. Finally, the aim of Phase III trials is explicitly to look at clinical outcomes – does the drug do what it's designed to do? All these factors, along with the randomised and blinded nature of these trials, add to the degree of confidence in the results.

So, in general the conclusion is that data from large Phase III trials is preferred to the data from earlier phase trials. But, unfortunately, there are often different Phase III trials looking at the same treatment in very similar circumstances in similar groups of patients. And, inevitably, it is not unusual to find that different Phase III trials can come to different conclusions. Despite the best efforts of all involved, even large trials can be subject to biases or poor design. Having a second, third or more Phase III trials looking at a drug or other treatment is a necessary step to show that good results can be replicated. In many cases replicating good results in additional Phase III trials is a requisite for getting a new drug licensed – though this is less of an issue in cancer than it is in some chronic but not life-threatening illnesses.

For this reason, the highest level of evidence comes from what are called meta-analyses of clinical trial data. The idea is simple – the data from all of the studies is pooled together, assessed for quality and then a statistical determination of the overall result is made. The people doing the meta-analysis are normally experts in statistical analysis and have not been involved in the individual studies. The Cochrane Collaboration is an international body of independent experts who undertake many meta-analyses in medicine, not just in cancer. In some cases a meta-analysis will exclude data from trials which are deemed to be of poor quality or which are subject to biases that cannot be corrected for. More importantly, where different trials have used slightly different outcome measures (to be discussed later) a meta-analysis may convert the data into a standard form so that studies can be compared side by side.

We can conclude, therefore, that in terms of the degree of weight which we want to give to data, we can have the most confidence in a structured meta-analysis of the type carried out by the Cochrane Collaboration and the least to single case reports with low levels of supporting evidence.

## Trial Outcomes

Having established some ground rules that we can apply when looking at the different sources of human data relating to cancer treatments we next come to the question of interpreting specific results. Unfortunately this too is a process that is fraught with complexity as even within Phase II or Phase III trials there are numerous trial end-points which are commonly used. These end-points can cover biochemical metrics, quality of life measures, different survival and other outcomes yardsticks. In short there is not a *single* set of outputs that enable us to easily judge whether a given intervention is actually delivering clinically meaningful positive results.

Before we start looking at the individual measures a word about time measurements, which are largely the main points of interest in looking at outcomes. Generally trial results are about time measurements from *randomisation* to a specific end. By randomisation they mean the point at which a patient is selected for a specific treatment arm in the trial – treatment commences soon after this point. The time periods are most often reported in terms of the average number of months for the patients in that treatment arm. Mathematically speaking the word average can mean different things depending on how it's calculated. In daily life average is usually synonymous with the mean – you add up all the numbers and then divide this by the number of numbers. So, the mean of 2, 2, 5, 6 and 7 is 4.4, which feels reasonable. However, the mean of 2, 2, 5, 6 and 700 is 143 – the one big figure of 700 has skewed the average so that it doesn't really represent the rest of the numbers, which are closer to 4 than 143. It is precisely for this reason that a different form of average is used, which is the median figure – which is defined as the middle of the range of numbers. So, the median of 2, 2, 5, 6 and 7 is 5, and the median of 2, 2, 5, 6 and 700 is also 5, it's not influenced by extreme numbers at either end of the scale. In medical papers it's the median figure that is most often used as it is thought to be more representative of what most patients in the trial have experienced, but occasionally the mean figure is also quoted. If you see a paper that quotes figures in terms of mean rather than median then it is important to look at the range of values included to see if there are one or two outliers that have skewed the mean.

The single most important measure of clinical benefit when looking at clinical trial data is overall survival (often abbreviated to OS). This is defined as the length of time from randomisation for the trial to death, from any cause. The latter point is important because some treatments may be so toxic that patients are at an increased risk of death long after their treatment has ended and they have recovered from the original illness. Sometimes you may see results listed for cancer-specific survival which can miss an increased risk of death post-treatment. This is also a number that is imprecise because it is often hard to pin down why a patient has died – was it the cancer, or a long-standing illness made worse by treatment or something else? Therefore, the preferred measure is all-cause mortality – even if this includes people knocked down in traffic or other accidents. These would be assumed to be the same in patients who've had the new treatment *and* those in the standard of care or placebo group.

However, it is not always possible to report overall survival – it takes many years to gather the data, particularly in slow-growing cancers and requires large populations to give a result that isn't easily skewed by chance events. Therefore there are a range of other outcomes measures which are also used, and it is here that much confusion can arise as many of them sound remarkably similar and the differences between them are not always clear at first sight.

In some cancers in which many of the patients who are treated undergo complete response a slightly different metric is used: disease-free survival (DFS).

This measures the time from randomisation to tumour recurrence or death from any cause. In these cancers patients may have good long-term prognoses but some subsequently suffer from a recurrence many months or years after treatment has ended. For these diseases DFS is the preferred metric.

After OS progression-free survival (PFS) is probably the next most important outcome measure in the majority of cancers. It is used more often than OS and DFS as it can be reported earlier than OS and often doesn't need such a high population of patients to produce a statistically acceptable result. PFS is defined as the time from randomisation until disease progression or death. Note that this means that it also measures the degree of time patients experience tumour regression and stable disease, which are good measures of benefit directly relevant to patients. However, it can be tricky extrapolating from PFS to looking at longer term overall survival. In some cases there can be good PFS but these need not mean that patients have longer overall survival.

A related measure that is also sometimes used is time to progression (TTP) – this is the time from randomisation to disease progression, but it doesn't include deaths. This makes it subtly different to PFS, but it does measure tumour regressions and stable disease so it's still a useful metric.

Time to treatment failure (TTF) measures time from randomisation to the failure of a treatment for whatever reason. While it may seem that this is the same as TTP, the fact is that treatments can fail for reasons other than disease progression, for example because of unacceptable side effects or a patient decides to stop the treatment for personal reasons and so on. Generally the use of this figure is not used as often as PFS or TTP, but when it does it may be that the treatment is particularly toxic. When assessing a treatment that has been reported in terms of TTF then it is very important you understand why this figure was used and that you check on the reported rate and severity of side effects.

Event free survival (EFS) measures the period during which patients do not suffer from any of a set of defined events, which may include things like specific symptoms (bone pain from tumours, for example), disease progression or the discontinuation of treatment for whatever reason. Because so many different things can be included in the 'events', this is not as useful an end-point as PFS or OS.

There are still other outcome metrics which are used, though less frequently than the ones listed so far. For example time to next treatment (TTNT) is used sometimes to indicate how long a patient remains on a treatment, this isn't often used in cancer but in the case of a chronic disease like rheumatoid arthritis this is a number that is of considerable interest to patients.

## Response/Survival Rates

Finally, there is one other important metric which is unrelated to the duration of responses but which is of some importance when assessing the results from a clinical trial: the objective response rate (ORR). This measures the proportion of patients who showed *some benefit* from the treatment being trialled. The ORR is the number of patients who showed disease regression in response to the treatment – that is it includes both partial and complete responses – as a proportion of the total number treated. Note that while this is an important metric to indicate the anti-tumour effectiveness of a drug, it *does not include* patients who exhibited stable disease. In the case where a good number of patients experienced prolonged stable disease they would not show up in the ORR but it's a positive response all the same. They would however be included in the clinical benefit rate (CBR), which is often used in trials of metastatic or advanced disease. It is, of course, also important to also look at the PFS or TTP in this situation.

An additional and important measure of benefit is the hazard ratio (HR), which is often reported when comparing two treatments. Strictly speaking the hazard ratio defines the relative rates of particular events (the hazards, e.g. disease progression, heart attack, death) per unit of time for two distinct treatment populations. The hazards in a HR calculation do not necessarily correspond to death they could refer to other types of event, for example, the occurrence of specific side effects or other health events like heart attacks or stroke. Typically the HR is based on a statistical model such as a Cox proportional hazards model, and is often illustrated with a Kaplan-Meier survival curve, which shows the proportion of each treatment group in which the event has *not* taken place (e.g. patients have not died) over a set time period.

We can show a simple example to make this clearer. Let us assume that there are two treatment groups in a clinical trial, group A receive the standard of care treatment, and group B receive standard of care plus a new drug. If we plot the percentage of each group who are alive over a two year period we get a survival curve:

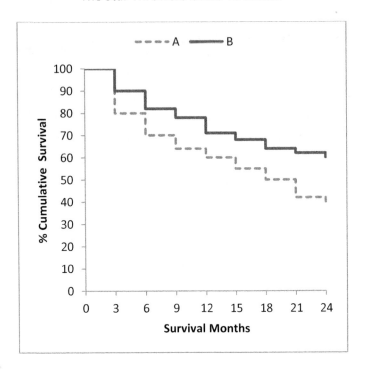

The graph illustrates that patients in group B, who had the new treatment, had better survival than the patients who had the standard treatment. At each time point we can see the percentage of patients who were alive in each group. The HR is related to this and gives us the ratio of risk in one group compared to another. A HR of 1 would mean that the risks are the same in each group, a HR greater than 1 says that there is a greater chance of an event occurring and a HR less than one is a reduced risk. In our example above, in which the chances of survival are greater at any time point in group B than in group A we would expect a HR of less than one (around 0.67 in fact – at any time point in the two years your chances are one third better of survival if you are in group B rather than in group B).

HR values are normally quoted with a 95% confidence interval, for example (HR=0.5, 95% CI 0.4 – 0.65). That is we are 95% certain that the real value for HR is in this range – and the reason we can't be 100% certain is that a clinical trial only includes a subset of the whole population of patients that might be treated, so there is a chance that if we had a different set of patients in the trial the actual numbers might have varied slightly. In general the more patients in a trial the more confident we can be in our results. This means that larger trials will have a much tighter band of values in the confidence interval than smaller trials.

An important metric that is used with HR and other statistics is the P-value, which is a measure of 'statistical significance'. This is a measure of confidence about the results and tells us something about the chance that the results could have come about by pure chance. Again, this is because in trials and experiments things are uncertain and results could be skewed by chance factors (for example your patients were particularly fit compared to the whole population of patients with that disease). A P-value of 0.05, also called the 5% value, suggests that there is a 1 in 20 chance that the result could have been down to chance. Normally a P value greater than 0.05 is considered non-significant, and a very low value of 0.01 or less is considered more significant – but keep in mind that these are statistical terms, not clinical. Statistical significance has become something of a fetish in the scientific world – there is nothing inherently special about the value of 0.05, it has just become something that is widely accepted.

Alongside the HR and P values it is always important to consider the clinical significance of what is being shown. Some clinical trials report excellent HR values and very good P values (P=0.0001), but the clinical significance is negligible – improvements of survival of a couple of weeks at the cost of severe side-effects and poor quality of life. Therefore, it is always essential to look at the clinical effect being reported, not just the statistical impressiveness.

## Summary

- Clinical research incudes data from human studies, particularly data from clinical trials
- Non-trial data can include case reports and data from analysis of historic results – this sort of data may be subject to all kinds of random biases, so is usually considered less definitive than data from prospective clinical trials
- Data from large Phase III randomised controlled trials is usually taken more seriously because the larger numbers of patients involved, and the use of a placebo or a comparison arm, mean that there is less chance (but not zero) of bias in the results
- Meta-analyses, where data from multiple trials are combined and then analysed together are the highest level of evidence of all in medicine
- When looking at results from trials it is important to take note of the response rates that are being used – overall survival and progression free survival are two of the most meaningful end points for studies and meta-analyses
- Statistical significance, commonly defined by a specific P-value (often 0.05), is not a measure of whether a result is medically important. It is a measure of confidence about the result – it is possible to be very confident about a result (for example

P=0.0001), but for the result to be of little clinical value

## References

1    Ezewuiro O, Grushko TA, Kocherginsky M, Habis M, et al. (2016) **Association of Metformin Use with Outcomes in Advanced Endometrial Cancer Treated with Chemotherapy.** *PloS one*, **11**(1), p. e0147145.

2    Chan AT, Arber N, Burn J, Chia WK, et al. (2012) **Aspirin in the chemoprevention of colorectal neoplasia: an overview.** *Cancer prevention research (Philadelphia, Pa.)*, **5**(2), pp. 164–78.

3    Forget P, Vandenhende J, Berliere M, MacHiels JP, et al. (2010) **Do intraoperative analgesics influence breast cancer recurrence after mastectomy? A retrospective analysis**. *Anesthesia and Analgesia*, **110**(6), pp. 1630–1635.

# Exploring Treatment Options Abroad

## Introduction

This chapter outlines the practical issues involved in gaining access to cancer treatments outside of the UK. It does not advocate for any particular treatment and does not recommend that cancer patients go abroad for treatment if there are equivalent treatment options available in this country. In particular, a great deal of caution needs to be exercised when looking at cancer treatments which have not been tested in clinical trials or which involve drugs or procedures not generally accepted in mainstream medicine.

However, with those caveats in mind there may be legitimate cause to seek medical treatment outside of the UK. Valid reasons may include:

- The lack of *any* viable treatment options in the UK and with no access to clinical trials possible (for further information on clinical trials please refer to the previous chapters on trials);
- The unavailability of specific interventions which have strong evidence of superior

239

outcomes in comparison to treatments available in the UK;

- The opportunity to participate in a clinical trial not available in the UK.

Before considering cancer treatment outside of the UK it is vitally important to do an analysis of the range of options available to you *in this country*. This may not be as straightforward as it should be. The NHS is a hugely complex structure with many local variations and areas of expertise scattered across the country. It is simply not always easy to discover if a specialist treatment is available or not. For example, some cancer ablation treatments, such as photodynamic therapy or radiofrequency ablation are only available in a few centres in the UK. It is sometimes easier to find a specialist offering these treatments outside of the UK than it is in the NHS, but they do exist here too (and are covered in the chapter on ablative treatments).

It is for this reason that the starting point for looking abroad has to be looking at home first. There are a number of strategies which can be adopted to make this task easier. The first and most obvious is to raise the issue with your existing oncologist or treatment team. Even if they are not convinced that the treatment you wish to explore is appropriate they may still be able to offer support in finding a suitably qualified specialist to make a referral to. Another good source is to look to patient self-help organisations or charities with particular areas of expertise. Check on good quality online forums dedicated to your particular cancer type. If the treatment is still considered experimental or an active area of research then use the PubMed database or Google Scholar to find doctors and scientists based in the UK who are active in that area.

If, after this period of research, the treatment you are seeking is not offered in the UK – and there is no other valid alternative – then it is time to explore accessing treatment abroad.

## Researching Treatments Abroad

There are numerous hospitals, clinics and doctors offering cancer treatments which are not available in the UK. There is a huge and sometimes bewildering range of treatments on offer. At one extreme there are treatments with new drugs, or medical technologies, not yet available in the UK, and that are firmly science-based and considered parts of 'conventional' medicine. At the other extreme there are those treatments that are decidedly unconventional and lacking credible scientific evidence. Unfortunately it is not always possible to clearly differentiate between the two, as increasingly there are unscrupulous individuals offering treatments which give a strong impression of being science-based, when in fact there is little solid evidence to support their use. It is a sad fact that there are many people, both inside the UK and abroad, who are more than happy to exploit desperate patients for financial gain.

While it is not the intention to survey the wide range of treatment options which are on offer abroad, it is perhaps instructive to look at three very specific cases of treatments which sound as though they are based on solid science when in fact the foundations are lacking and there are questions marks about the integrity of the people that offer them.

## Fake Science

The first is antineoplaston treatment, offered in the United States by the Burzynski Clinic in Houston, Texas. Discovered by Dr Stanislaw Burzynski, antineoplastons are described as naturally occurring biological molecules which have natural anticancer properties. They are said to re-programme cancer cells, whilst having low toxicity and are not harmful non-cancer cells. While antineoplastons are said to treat all forms of cancer, there is an emphasis on brain tumours in much of the marketing material produced by the Clinic. To all intents and purposes the marketing makes this sound like an ideal treatment option – non-toxic, delivered by scientists and doctors and said to treat even late stage cancers.

The reality is that the level of evidence for antineoplastons is very weak. The results that the Clinic claims for the treatments have not been independently verified. While numerous clinical trials have been initiated by the Clinic, these are seldom completed and are seen primarily as a means for the clinic to by-pass regulations which prohibit unlicensed treatments except in the case of clinical trials. Extensive use is made of anecdotes and patient stories in a bid to convince would-be patients that this is a viable option. While some research papers are published, these are not published in reputable journals, and do not include the rigorous analysis which would convince most doctors. Much of the published research is about laboratory cell lines rather than human data from clinical trials. What is more the treatment is expensive, can be extremely toxic and frequently will include many of the standard chemotherapy drugs which proponents of antineoplastons criticise. In short, the Burzynski clinic uses the trappings of science as a marketing tool and offers an untested and *potentially very dangerous* treatment at great financial cost.

Closer to home, a similar use of the trappings of science surrounds the use of GcMAF. Like antineoplastons, there are numerous claims made about the efficacy of this protein, not just against cancer but against a wide range of conditions, including autism, chronic fatigue syndrome, Alzheimer's, multiple sclerosis and more. It is claimed that GcMAF is 'the body's internal medicine' and that it 'directs the immune system' to destroy cancer. Treatment with GcMAF can take place at a number of clinics abroad, but it is also aggressively sold over the internet so that people can self-treat. As with antineoplastons, much is made of the non-toxic, natural and safe nature of the treatment in contrast to the rigours of chemotherapy and radiotherapy. And, again, much is made of the 'science'. The people selling GcMAF make much of the numerous papers published in peer reviewed oncology journals. As with antineoplastons much of this research is based on in vitro studies in cell lines and not based on human data.

From the outside this does appear to be scientifically based. But the fact is that there have been no clinical trials to show whether GcMAF works or not. There is no independent verification of the cases that are mentioned on the internet sites which promote or sell GcMAF. Many of the papers are of poor quality and some are published in fake journals (also known as 'predatory journals' in the science community). A number of these papers have since been withdrawn as investigators, such as the Belgian Anticancer Fund, have shown that the data is faked or suspect. Like the Burzynski case, this too is more about making money from desperate patients than it is about research or proving that there really is something to GcMAF.

The final example is not based on a drug but on a treatment technique called sonodynamic therapy (SDT), also sometimes called Next Generation Photodynamic Therapy (NGPDT). Photodynamic Therapy (PDT) is a treatment technique that involves the injection of a light-sensitive dye, called a photosensitiser drug, into patients. This drug accumulates more in tumour cells than in non-cancer cells and is designed to react when it comes into contact with certain frequencies of light. Patients who have been injected with the dye must stay out of the light while the drug is active. After the drug has been allowed to accumulate in the tumour a surgeon will apply a laser or other light source to the tumour. Often a surgeon will have to make an incision so that the light source can be brought into close contact with tumours below the surface of the skin. When the drug comes into contact with the light it reacts, releasing very volatile molecules which can destroy the tumour cells. PDT is available on the NHS, but is not widely used throughout the country. SDT and NGPDT treatments are offered in a small number of private clinics in the UK and more widely abroad.

SDT and NGPDT claim to be based on similar principles to basic PDT. Patients have to take a sensitiser drug which accumulates in tumour tissues, and after this has happened a treatment takes place which causes the drug to react and hence kill the tumour cells. In the case of SDT and NGPDT there is little evidence that the treatments work as they are said to. For example there is no evidence that light sources used in NGPDT can penetrate more than a few millimetres below the surface of the skin – often a light-bed is used and no surgical incisions are made to gain access to deep-seated tumour tissues. In the case of SDT ultrasound is also used, but again there is no evidence that this is effective. As with the previous examples, much is made of the scientific and technological evidence for these treatments in a bid to convince patients that they are accessing something with evidence of efficacy, but no solid clinical trials have shown that these treatments work. Again, there is no independently verified clinical trial data to back up the extraordinary claims made for this 'treatment'.

What all of these examples have in common is that they are sold to patients using the language of science, with papers in journals and technical jargon to back them up, but this is just clever marketing aimed at disarming the sceptical but desperate patient. Like other such examples they make extravagant promises of excellent results (including miraculous cases in late stage cancers), make a big play about lack of toxicity or using the body's own defences and they come with significant financial costs. Additionally, the people marketing these treatments will frequently encourage a conspiratorial view of medicine – they will claim that the truth of their miraculous results is being suppressed by the pharmaceutical companies or by oncologists or governments. They will point to their conflicts with regulators as evidence for these conspiracies, though in truth patient safety concerns is the more obvious reason to explain conflicts with authority.

The bottom line for patients seeking science-based treatments abroad is that scientific language and a set of technical articles is not enough. Warning bells should be triggered whenever you see a promise of miraculous results, and these warning bells should rise to an absolute clamour should the treatment that produces these miracles be described as risk-free, 'natural' or suppressed by the mainstream.

A checklist of questions to help assess the trustworthiness of a proposed cancer treatment is included below.

## 'Alternative Medicine'

Another class of treatment that are frequently offered abroad are the 'alternative medicine' treatments which do not attempt to deploy the language or trappings of conventional medical science. Frequently these treatments make a virtue of out-right rejection of conventional medicine and instead will be based on homeopathy, special diets, spiritual healing and so on. While there is some evidence that things like Reiki and other interventions can have positive effects on mood, stress-levels and mental well-being, there is no evidence that these treatments have a clinical effect on cancer. They can certainly be used as *complementary* treatments alongside conventional treatments. However, any 'alternative' clinic that recommends that standard treatments *should not be* used by patients, especially newly-diagnosed patients, **should be avoided at all costs**. While standard treatments are often toxic, dangerous and not as effective as we would like, they remain superior to untested and unscientific therapies with no real evidence of effect.

## A Checklist for Treatments Abroad

The following list of questions may be useful when assessing whether a treatment offered abroad is trustworthy enough to investigate further:

- Is there high-quality published evidence in favour of this treatment? The highest quality evidence would be in the form of results from a registered clinical trial published in a respected peer-reviewed journal. Case series or individual case reports are also useful but not as important as trial data. Be aware that some 'scientific journals' are fake (these are known as predatory journals) and they are designed to scam scientists and members of the public alike. Some fake cancer cures are using these predatory journals to publish 'data' which show miraculous cancer cures. Please cross-check the journal with the list of predatory journals maintained on the http://scholarlyoa.com/ website.

- Is it clear where the treatment will take place, who will be administering the treatment and what the treatment actually involves? Have the potential side-effects, both the severity and duration, been discussed? Will the clinic include after-care following the administration of drugs, surgery or other treatment?

- Are the people who will administer the treatment suitably qualified? Be aware that the title Dr can describe both medical practitioners (an M.D.) and people who have studied for a doctorate (a Ph.D.). If the person has a Ph.D. and is not a qualified medical practitioner then this should raise alarm. No suitably qualified clinician will object if you ask for verification of qualifications.

- Have the people who will administer the treatment asked you the right questions? Have they asked in detail about your medical history, your diagnosis and current treatments? Have they requested access to medical records or scans? Have they asked about your current physical status or are they more interested in your financial arrangements?

- When communicating with the clinic have you established that there are no language issues? Be aware that many of the clinics in non-English and non-European countries employ people who have excellent language skills to talk to patients and potential patients, but that these are not the people administering the treatments. In your communications it is important that you speak directly with the clinicians, not just the administrative and financial staff.

- Have you established that they have experience with your specific diagnosis and stage of disease? Cancer is many diseases, and breast cancer is actually a family of different diseases with different treatment options depending on sub-type and staging. In the case of metastatic disease there are enormous differences between dealing with bone disease compared to lung or liver for example. You need to be certain that they have the appropriate expertise for your specific condition – how many times have they treated, when was the last time etc.

- Is the clinic or treatment licensed or regulated or does it exist outside of the local health system in the country in which you are seeking treatment? The Health Regulation Worldwide website (http://www.healthregulation.org/) lists regulators for different specialisms across the world.

- It is strongly advised that you speak to other patients who have been treated and/or have received the specific treatment that you are interested in. If the clinic does not support you in doing this then it is *not* a good sign. There are numerous patient forums available online – it is also advised that you search these for evidence from previous patients. You may also want to post a message to such forums and ask for experiences yourself.

- How will the success of the treatment be assessed? Where and when will this assessment take place? Will it be included in the costs of the treatment or is this additional?

- If the treatment involves surgery or other invasive procedure, toxic drugs (e.g. chemotherapy) or other potentially dangerous intervention, does the clinic have appropriate emergency facilities and staff to deal with it?
- Will the clinic supply medical notes, scans and full details of your treatment and condition to your oncology team back in the UK? Will there be additional costs for this documentation?

This list is by no means exhaustive but it includes many of the most important questions to ask – at the very least it will establish a detailed dialogue with the clinic or clinician. How they respond will be as important as some of the individual answers – you will need to feel that you can trust the people you are dealing with. However, be aware that there are some very slick operations in existence and they are adept at dealing with people – this is one reason that it is so essential that you seek independent verification of all claims. As always be aware of people promising miraculous results – even with the most promising treatments there are so many variables involved that an honest clinician will always remain cautious. *In particular it is important to have some independent contact with previous patients.*

### Getting a Second Opinion

If, after having done your research, including working through the above set of questions, you have identified a treatment that you feel is appropriate for your situation, it is important to get a second opinion. Ideally this second opinion should come from your existing doctors, preferably from your existing oncology team or your GP. It is possible, even likely, that they will not support your decision but it is important that you understand their reasoning. Is there something specific about the treatment? Is it a concern about the individuals who will be treating you? It may simply be a concern that your proposed treatment may impose a significant strain on your current physical condition. It is also possible that they will engage with the clinicians abroad directly, or possibly they will ask that you ensure you come back with any scans, x-rays, blood results and medical notes.

In any event, you need to understand the particular concerns they express. You may assess these concerns and decide that you want to proceed – as is your right – or you may want to amend your plans. In either case you will return to the UK after you have had treatment abroad, and your doctors will need to understand where you have been and what treatment you have had.

It may also be worth getting a second opinion from support groups or charities which help people with your specific diagnosis, or a group like Star Throwers which supports late-stage cancer patients.

## Funding Treatments Abroad

*Note that at the time of publication these rules are still in place – but with the 2016 vote to leave the European Union it is not clear how things will change in the future.*

Inevitably, cost is a big factor in looking at treatments abroad. There are some options for seeking funding from the NHS for *some* treatments in *some* European countries. Firstly, this funding is only available to countries within the European Economic Area (EEA) – this includes all of the EU countries, with the addition of Iceland, Norway and Liechtenstein, and, in some circumstances, Switzerland. This is not to say that it is not possible to get funding for treatment in the USA or other countries not in the EEA; it is, but the process is more complex and less likely to succeed. In the first instance, should you want to explore funding for treatment in a non-EEA country, then you have to contact your local NHS Clinical Commissioning Group.

For treatment in EEA countries there are two possible funding mechanisms, but both apply to treatment in the state systems – which in some countries may also include private clinics. Each country publishes a web-site which lists the available treatments – and the list of these sites can be downloaded here: http://ec.europa.eu/health/cross_border_care/docs/cb hc_ncp_en.pdf. These national contact sites link to search engines which you can use to check whether the clinic you have identified is included. Of course it is also possible to start your search for treatment abroad by looking through these sites. Note that different countries have different rules over what is or is not included in their state systems; so it is possible to find that treatments not available in the UK are included in other countries, but this does not necessarily mean that you will be able to access them – that depends on NHS approval.

The two funding mechanisms available for EEA countries are called the S2 route or the EU Directive route. In neither case does funding cover travel, insurance or additional accommodation costs. The main differences between these options revolves around methods of payment – does the NHS pay or does the patient pay and then claim it back from the NHS?

The S2 route means that payment for the treatment is arranged between the NHS and the health provider in the other country. Prior agreement is required for this, and the NHS publishes an extensive list of the conditions which are covered here: http://www.nhs.uk/NHSEngland/Healthcareabroad/p lannedtreatment/Documents/services-subject-to-prior-authorisation.pdf. Note that it *does* include specialist cancer care for both adults and children/adolescents. Approval is dependent on a number of conditions:

- Written approval from a UK consultant that the treatment is warranted and that a full clinical assessment of possible benefit has been carried out
- That the local NHS Commissioner agrees that the costs are justified
- That the patient is eligible for NHS treatment and that the treatment abroad falls within the remit of the scheme

Note that the payments levied for the treatment are the same as that charged to local patients in that country – this may mean that only a portion of the treatment costs are covered and that this will have to be 'topped up' by the you directly. These 'top up' costs may be reimbursed when you return to the UK by applying to the NHS. The application form for prior authorisation can be downloaded via http://www.nhs.uk/NHSEngland/Healthcareabroad/plannedtreatment/Pages/TheE112.aspx.

The EU Directive route differs from the S2 route in that the patient pays for the treatment directly and then has to claim reimbursement on returning to the UK. Because of this there is some additional flexibility in that it can include some private clinics and other providers outside of the state system in each country. As with the S2 route it is highly recommended that you pre-authorise treatment so that you can be certain that some or all of your costs will be reimbursed. The rules for which treatments apply are relatively straightforward; it covers costs for treatments which are available in the NHS. There are some cases where there is an unacceptably long waiting period for a treatment which is available more quickly abroad, in such situations this route can speed things along.

The application form for the EU directive route can be downloaded via http://www.nhs.uk/NHSEngland/Healthcareabroad/plannedtreatment/Pages/Article56.aspx.

## Summary

- Before seeking specific treatments abroad it is important to check whether the treatment is already available in the UK. Often there are promising treatments which are available in the UK but only in a few centres
- Good research is absolutely essential when seeking new options abroad. While there are promising and novel treatments on offer in some other countries, there are also many people offering untested, unscientific or dangerous treatments
- Some scammers are deliberately seeking to exploit vulnerable cancer patients by promising miraculous cures. Many of them are using the trappings of science so that they appear credible and genuine, so extra care must be taken to verify all claims
- Use the checklist of questions in this document to ascertain whether the treatments offered are worth following up or not. At the very least it will help you gauge the level of trust and transparency
- It is important to try and learn from existing or previous patients who have used the clinic or treatment being offered
- Always get a second opinion on a treatment that you find abroad
- Make sure you inform your existing medical team – if possible get their opinion and involvement

- Treatments within the European Economic Area (EEA) can be refunded by the NHS. But only for specific treatments and with the sign-off from your NHS consultant. It is best practice to always pre-authorise any treatments for which you will seek funding or reimbursement

- The S2 funding route means the NHS pays the state health provider in the country offering the treatment. Some costs may have to be paid by the patient, but these may be eligible for reimbursement by the NHS

- The EU Directive route means the patient pays for the treatment and is then reimbursed on returning to the UK. This route has greater flexibility in terms of service providers but as with the other route it is advisable to get pre-authorisation

- NHS funding of treatments in all other countries have to be applied for on a case by case basis

# Ablative Therapies

## Introduction

Normally we think of surgery, radiotherapy and chemotherapy as the standard treatments for cancer, but increasingly these are being joined by a diverse set of treatments that are used to directly attack tumour masses. Using a variety of technologies, these treatments can be grouped together as 'ablative therapies' in that they physically remove or destroy cancerous and non-cancerous growths. The word 'ablation' actually means the loss, or removal, of a part – for example the loss of ice from a glacier. In this case we are talking about non-surgical treatments that physically remove all or part of a tumour. Examples include photodynamic therapy (PDT), radiofrequency ablation (RFA), cryoablation and so-called 'nanoknife' treatments. This chapter will introduce each of these treatments and outline how they work, which cancers they apply to and the specific situations in which they are used.

It should be noted at the outset that unlike chemotherapy, these are not 'systemic' treatments. That is they are not used to treat the whole body, in that sense they are not like chemotherapy which can target tumours wherever they are located. Instead these are considered 'local treatments' in that they target tumours at specific sites. Oncologists will sometimes term this a 'focal' treatment – particularly in the case of prostate cancer where such treatments are becoming increasingly important. That is not to say that such treatments cannot have a systemic effect, as we will see there is some evidence that some of these treatments can invoke immune responses which will act throughout the body, but when this happens it is considered a positive by-product rather than an intrinsic part of the treatment plan.

Unlike the big three of surgery, radiotherapy and chemotherapy, access to these treatments is not always easy in the UK. Provision is extremely patchy and varies across the country, but in general this is an improving picture. In part, this process of increasing provision is driven by positive results from clinical trials, but it is also true that these treatments are generally considered very cost effective. Ablative treatments tend to be relatively quick to administer and to have faster recovery times than surgical interventions which are often the main alternative for treating localised disease. Given that, it is also true that it is often the case that oncologists themselves are not aware of the range of treatments on offer or of their availability in the NHS. In such circumstances it makes sense for patients to investigate the availability themselves, and where possible points of contact are provided to help the reader access relevant information themselves.

## Photodynamic Therapy (PDT)

PDT is a treatment that uses a class of drug called a photosensitiser together with the application of light to destroy tumour tissues. Although there are different types of PDT in use, with very different treatment procedures in practice, all work on the same underlying principle. First the photosensitive drug is applied directly to – or absorbed by – the tissues to be treated, and then particular wavelengths of light are applied. The photosensitive drug reacts to the light by producing highly reactive oxygen molecules which destroy the cells they are in contact with, thereby directly killing the tissues or tumours which contain the drug.

PDT is used to treat a variety of conditions, not just cancer. For example it is used to treat a range of skin conditions including severe acne, rosacea, warts and other non-cancerous skin lesions. In this form of PDT the photosensitiser is applied directly to the skin which is to be treated and then, after a suitable period in which the drug is absorbed by the lesion, light of a specific wavelength is applied via a laser or LED. The drug reacts to the light and the lesion is effectively destroyed. Some forms of non-melanoma skin cancer are treated in this way, though only superficial lesions can be treated as the light sources cannot penetrate more than a centimetre below the surface of the skin.

In the case of using PDT for cancer, the procedure is generally more complex. Firstly the photosensitiser is normally administered intravenously and circulates via the blood stream to tissues and organs throughout the body. The drug accumulates preferentially in tumour cells, though some will also be absorbed by non-tumour cells. Typically there is a waiting period – often called the incubation period – of between two to four days to ensure that as much of the drug accumulates in the tumour as possible. During this incubation period the patient has to be cautious about exposure to light, which will react with the photosensitiser that is still circulating or is absorbed by non-cancer tissues. Typically the patient has to remain in a darkened room, wear sunglasses and generally be very wary of accidental exposure to light.

Because PDT depends on the application of a light source it is mainly used for cancers which are not in deep-seated or hard to access sites. The main cancers treated in this way are non-melanoma skin cancers (such as basal cell carcinoma), head and neck cancers, oesophageal cancer and some tumours in the lungs. There have also been trials of PDT in a wide range of other cancers, including breast, colorectal, glioblastoma, cholangiocarcinoma, prostate and other cancers. There are numerous active clinical trials of PDT in a broad range of cancers currently on-going, and patients who are interested in exploring this option should refer to the chapter on searching for clinical trials for details on how to look for appropriate trials.

The light sources used for PDT are tuned to deliver just the right frequency of light to trigger the reaction from the photosensitive drug. The light has to be brought into very close contact with the tumours or tissues to be treated, which often means that the patient has to take a local or general anaesthetic during the procedure. Access is often via the mouth or nose and involves the insertion of fibre optic cables to deliver the light to the tumour – sometimes ultrasound or MRI is used to guide the fibre optics into place. Larger tumours may be treated using interstitial PDT which involves the fibre optics being inserted directly into the tumours before the light is applied.

PDT has the advantage that the treatment can be repeated multiple times, unlike radiotherapy or surgery. Treatment times are also generally shorter than surgery – typical treatment times are less than an hour. However, there is a downside in that there is still a recovery period required, during which patients are sensitive to light. Generally patients have to take precautions to avoid exposure to direct sunlight for around two weeks if the IV form of photosensitiser has been used (which it normally is for non-skin cancers). Common side effects include residual photosensitivity, which subsides with time, localised pain at the treatment site and a risk of infection.

It is important to note that PDT is generally viewed as a tool for local control of tumour growth. As such it is often used to 'debulk' tumours to clear airways or to address specific problems caused by locally active tumour growth. It is not generally viewed as a curative treatment, although there are patients who do achieve long-term remissions.

In addition to the local destruction of cancer cells by reactive oxygen molecules, it is thought that PDT also works through two additional mechanisms. The first is by destroying the blood vessels which feed nutrients and oxygen to the tumours – effectively cutting off one of the main supply routes into the tumour mass. Secondly the killing of the tumour cells can mobilise an immune response, which kicks in and accelerates the destruction of the tumour. The good news is that the immune response can be systemic, (in which case it is described as an *abscopal* response), and in theory other tumours in the body, which have not been treated with PDT, will also suffer the immune response. Unfortunately there is still much that we do not understand about how to maximise this systemic effect and currently there are no standard mechanisms in place with which to strengthen this immune response.

There is much active research on PDT, looking both at new and more powerful photosensitising drugs and also at extending the range of cancers in which it is used. Important strands of research are also looking at how PDT can be combined with other treatments to maximise the benefits that it brings. One alluring prospect – which has yet to be explored clinically – is the combination of PDT and metronomic chemotherapy (covered in a separate chapter), or the combination of PDT and non-cancer drugs which impact the microenvironment which provide the support systems that tumours need to survive and prosper.

Mention must be made of so-called 'Next Generation PDT' and 'Sonodynamic Therapy' – these are treatments which are offered in a number of private clinics here in the UK and abroad. There are numerous extravagant claims made for these treatments (discussed also in the chapter on treatments abroad). For example that they can treat deep-seated tumours without the need to gain access to the tumours directly, or that patients can sit under a sun-bed and be treated for widely spread disease deep below the surface of the skin. These claims are designed deliberately to exploit vulnerable and desperate people. There is no scientific basis for many of these claims, and there have been no clinical trials or studies to show that these 'treatments' actually work at all. While there have been some test tube and animal experiments using sonodynamic therapy (which combines sound and light), there has not been a single trial ever registered for it. Effectively these are scams designed to steal money from desperate people looking for a miracle – it is strongly advised that you avoid any clinics or doctors who offer these fake treatments as they are not to be trusted.

The best place to discover the range of PDT treatments and trials on offer in the UK is via the charity Killing Cancer (www.killingcancer.co.uk).

## Radiofrequency Ablation (RFA)

Where PDT uses the delivery of light to tumours, RFA uses the delivery of electrical energy to generate heat to destroy cancer tissues. Together with microwave ablation, RFA is classed as a thermal ablation treatment because it's ultimately the heat that is generated which kills the tumour cells. As with the other ablative therapies, RFA is a local treatment in that it is used to target specific tumour masses rather than a systemic treatment that can treat the whole body or large areas. This does not necessarily mean that only one tumour at a time can be treated, it is possible to treat multiple tumours within a single treatment session, but each must be treated directly.

Treatment consists of the insertion of very thin needle-like probes into the tumour tissue followed by the application of a high-frequency electrical signal. This generates high levels of heat at the very tip of the probe, and it is this heat which effectively kills the tumour. The heat produced is very localised and does not cause widespread burns, nor does the electrical energy that produces the heat cause electric shocks – indeed RFA is considered to be a very safe treatment type. The clinician administering the treatment will use ultrasound or other imaging to help guide the probes into the tumour masses. Mostly the procedure is performed under a general anaesthetic, but sometimes the patient will have received a local anaesthetic and will be awake during the procedure. In some cases the treatment may be performed at the same time as surgery or a laparoscopy. More than one probe can be used and, in larger tumours, several may be inserted into the same mass in a single treatment session. A typical treatment lasts between 60 – 90 minutes depending on the number of tumours and the complexity of the treatment plan.

Note than in contrast to PDT it is possible to use RFA to treat deep-seated tumours, and it is most often used to treat tumours in the lungs (both primary tumours and metastases), the liver (primaries and metastases), kidney cancer and oesophageal cancer. It has been used to treat some benign bone tumours and other conditions, and there is active research looking at using RFA for a broader range of cancers, including breast, prostate, pancreatic, colorectal and some sarcomas.

Because the heat generated by RFA is very localised there are limits to the size of tumours that can be treated, even when multiple probes are used. The sizes vary by tumour site and also by the number of tumours that need to be treated. For example current guidelines for lung tumours are that there should be fewer than 5 tumours per lung and that these should be less than 3.5 cm in diameter. Only one lung can be treated at a time. Slightly different rules apply for liver and other sites. However, there is obviously variation among patients and there is flexibility in drawing up treatment plans.

As with all forms of treatment there are side effects, which include local inflammation and pain at the treatment site. Some patients experience fatigue and a general 'under the weather' feeling, possibly due to the immune reaction that is provoked by the treatment. However, the side effects are rarely serious and most patients do not require a hospital stay after treatment, unless it is combined with surgery or other treatment.

In addition to exploring the use of RFA in new cancer types, there is active research to understand whether combination treatments provide the best response. For example does the combination of RFA and the chemotherapy drug sorafenib work better than either treatment alone? Similarly there is active research to find ways of potentiating the systemic immune response that treatment induces. The hope is that if the immune response can be potentiated then local RFA treatments will have effects on distant untreated tumours.

While RFA is an established treatment choice there are many oncologists who do not routinely suggest it to their patients. It is available at a number of centres in the UK, and many of these will accept referrals from other areas which do not offer this treatment. A good starting place for anyone wanting to explore this treatment option is The Cancer Thermal Ablation Fund (http://www.rfablation.co.uk), which is a small charity that provides information and advice to patients.

## Microwave Ablation (MWA)

In most respects this is the same as RFA except that the frequencies used are much higher and the temperature produced at the tip of the probe is also correspondingly higher. Tumour kill is still due to the intense heat effectively burning the cancer cells. The heat is still localised however, and a typical treatment will use multiple probes to target the tumour. MWA is a newer treatment than RFA and is used to treat many of the same cancer types. The safety profile and side effects are also very similar – though there is some evidence that RFA may have a slightly better safety profile than MWA. In terms of providing better outcomes the evidence is inconclusive at the moment, although there have been some small trials which show a marginal reduction in recurrence rates for MWA compared to RFA. Many of the centres which offer RFA also offer MWA, and the choice of treatment will be made by a multidisciplinary team meeting based on the specifics of a patient's case.

As a relatively new treatment there is still much active research on MWA, both to extend the range of cancer types that it is used for, and also to identify which other treatments it is best combined with. There are numerous clinical trials on-going and so it is worth investigating these should you be interested in this treatment type.

There are numerous centres available in the UK, both on the NHS and private clinics, which offer MWA. The Cancer Thermal Ablation Fund (http://www.rfablation.co.uk) is a good source of information and may help in identifying a suitable centre that is local to your area.

## Cryoablation (CA)

Where RFA and MWA generate heat to attack tumours, cryoablation takes the opposite approach and generates very low temperatures to freeze and kill cancer cells. Also known as cryotherapy or cryosurgery, CA is another treatment that acts on localised tumours rather than systemic disease. The treatment can be administered under local anaesthetic or sedative, but it is more frequently used when the patient has taken a general anaesthetic. Very fine hollow needles are inserted into the tumours, usually under CT or ultrasound guidance, and then ice-cold gas or fluid is pumped into the tissues. This causes ice to form in the affected tissues, thereby killing cells in the immediate vicinity. Repeated cycles of freezing and thawing are used to maximise the rate of tumour kill – with imaging used to monitor the growth of the 'ice ball' during the treatment. The ice ball is sustained for around 10 -15 minutes to guarantee that cells die – both by ice formation inside the cancer cells and also by the freezing of the blood supply into the tumour.

A range of cancers can be treated using CA, including early stage prostate and kidney cancers, tumours in the lungs and liver, pediatric retinoblastomas and some breast cancers. It has also been used to treat pain associated with metastatic disease in the bones. As with the other ablative therapies listed above, there is much active research to assess the long-term benefits of CA in comparison to surgery and other treatments, and also to investigate the use of the treatment in a wider range of cancer types. There are numerous on-going clinical trials listed in the main trial registries and anyone interested in this option is advised to look for a suitable trial in the first instance.

Side-effects are similar to RFA and MWA, and include damage to adjacent tissues, local inflammation and a general 'under the weather' feeling as the immune system copes with the effect of the dead cancer tissue. Additionally, cryoablation carries the risk of nerve damage when the ice ball also includes nerve cells within it.

While CA is available at a number of different centres in the UK, there is no central point of contact devoted to this treatment modality. The Cancer Thermal Ablation Fund (http://www.rfablation.co.uk) has some coverage of CA, as does the Interventional Oncology Service based at University College London Hospital (http://www.uclh.nhs.uk/OurServices/ServiceA-Z/IMAGING/IOS/Pages/Home.aspx).

## Irreversible Electroporation (IRE)

Also known as Nanoknife therapy, irreversible electroporation is another ablative therapy for treating localised tumours. The treatment works by applying electric fields to tumour cells – in other words electrocuting cancer cells rather than heating or freezing them. The high-voltage electric field creates tiny holes (pores) in the cancer cells which cause the cells to die – the holes in the cell walls cannot be repaired hence the term 'irreversible electroporation'. Because the effect is due to the electric field rather than due to the creation of heat energy there is little in the way of collateral damage to adjacent tissues.

As with many of the other treatments outlined in this chapter, IRE is primarily a percutaneous (through the skin) treatment. It can also be used via laparoscopy (a small incision in the abdomen allowing access to internal organs) or with other surgical intervention. The treatment is applied via needle-like electrodes passed through the skin to the target tissues to be treated. A typical treatment may use a number of these electrodes at any one time. High-voltage DC electricity is applied via the electrodes in very short pulses of around 100 ms and between 90 and 100 pulses are used in a typical treatment. The patient is generally treated under general anaesthetic, and CT or other imaging is used to guide the treatment.

The area affected by the field is generally very constrained and there is less damage to adjacent tissues than is the case with some of the other ablation techniques. In terms of pain and side effects the evidence to date suggests a very good safety profile and that the post-operative pain is comparable to that experienced with RFA. A particular advantage of IRE compared to thermal or cryoablation is that it preserves tissues such as blood vessels and bile ducts, making treatment of tumours close to major blood vessels feasible. This is particularly important in the case of liver and pancreatic tumours.

In terms of cancer types treated, the range is similar to the other ablative interventions: liver tumours (primary and metastatic), tumours in the lungs and pancreas. It has also been used in animal models of cancers of the kidney, breast, cervical, prostate, and brain, as well as soft tissue and bone sarcomas. Some of these animal experiments are being followed up in clinical trials in humans, with a good number of trials currently open to recruitment in a range of cancer types.

Unlike the other ablative therapies outlined previously there is less evidence that IRE provokes a systemic immune response – in part this is presumed to be due to the different way that IRE kills cells – through the process of apoptosis rather than the necrosis caused by heating or freezing cells. However, this is less of an issue in cancer patients who have compromised immune systems and therefore not in the best state to mount an immune response – even when one is provoked by high degrees of necrotic cell death.

As a relatively new treatment, (the first commercial equipment for IRE, the Nanoknife system, was only licensed in 2007), IRE is the subject of intense research. Not only in exploring the efficacy of it compared to other treatments, or in extending the use to new cancers, but also in improving the existing treatment. For example, there is research looking at the use of different electrode designs, in exploring the use of alternating current rather than DC and in how best to combine it with chemotherapy and other treatments.

IRE is becoming more widely used and is available in multiple centres in the UK via the NHS, as well as in some private clinics. There is no central contact point for IRE, however, and finding a local centre that provides the treatment may necessitate some internet searching. The UCLH Interventional Oncology Service may also be of some use for those patients looking for a referral to a centre with wide experience using IRE.

# High Intensity Focused Ultrasound (HIFU)

The final ablative therapy we will explore is based on the use of specialised ultrasound equipment. This is used to focus high-frequency sound waves onto specifically targeted tissues, in order to kill cancer cells. HIFU is not yet in general use in the NHS, but it is available in some centres via clinical trials and also in some private clinics in the UK. The most advanced work on this is in the treatment of prostate cancer, but there are also trials in the UK in some other cancers, including bone metastases and pancreatic and liver cancers.

HIFU treatment for prostate cancer is carried out under a general anaesthetic and involves the insertion of an ultrasound probe, via the rectum, to a position close to the prostate. Ultrasound is then applied and this has the effect of heating up the surrounding tissue and killing the cancer cells. The procedure has shown positive results in some small trials in the UK and some larger trials in other countries. Compared to some other treatments for localised prostate cancer the safety profile is very good, and patients do not suffer as many side effects with respect to erectile dysfunction and urinary incontinence.

There is no central point of contact in the UK for HIFU treatments. The treatment is available on the NHS in some hospitals, and also at a number of private clinics. If you are interested in this treatment option the first port of call should be your oncologist who can help identify a practitioner. Alternatively you may want to contact the University College London Hospital Prostate Cancer Team https://www.uclh.nhs.uk/OurServices/ServiceA-Z/Cancer/UROCAN/PROSTCAN/Pages/Treatingpro statecancer.aspx.

## Summary

- Ablative therapies are a collection of treatments which target specific tumour masses, rather than being available for systemic treatment of widely disseminated disease
- These treatments are often used in a palliative setting or used to achieve local control of cancer
- Photodynamic therapy involves the administration of a light sensitive drug which reacts when a specific frequency of light is applied to it. The chemical reaction between the drug and the light creates very reactive molecules which kill the affected cells
- Radiofrequency and microwave ablation use the targeted application of heat energy to

raise the temperature of the tumour tissues being treated so that cancer cells in the immediate vicinity are killed
- Cryoablation takes a similar approach except that it uses extreme cold to kill the target cells, not heat
- Irreversible electroporation applies high-power pulses of electric current to irreparably damage the target cells
- High intensity focused ultrasound applies very focused sound waves to heat up the target tissues and kill cells

# Metronomic Chemotherapy

## Introduction

Chemotherapy is a mainstay of cancer treatment – and has been for decades now, despite advances in other forms of treatment. It is also the treatment that patients dread the most because of the frequent and debilitating side effects associated with it. In this article we will explore the rationale behind chemotherapy, look at the causes of these side effects and then consider an alternative approach to treatment that utilises many of the same chemotherapeutic drugs but in a radically different way. This alternative approach is called metronomic chemotherapy, and although it may sound similar to the standard treatment approach, it is in fact a very different concept altogether and may be a viable option in some late stage cancers.

## A History Lesson

Before we can understand the differences between standard chemotherapy and the low-dose metronomic alternative it is instructive to learn a little about how the standard practice *became* the standard. This historical detour begins in the early

1940s in the United States, with a project by the Department of Defence to examine the therapeutic potential of a number of chemical warfare agents. In 1942 two pharmacologists, Louis Goodman and Alfred Gilman persuaded Gustav Lindskog, a thoracic surgeon, to treat a patient with non-Hodgkin's lymphoma with nitrogen mustard (similar to the poison gas used in the First World War). This produced a profound but short-lived regression in the tumours, the first time a chemical had been shown to have such an effect in human cancers. Later, in 1948, Sydney Farber and colleagues worked on a new class of drugs called anti-folates which they prescribed to children suffering from acute lymphoblastic leukaemia (ALL). Again, there were remissions in patients, although not long-term. It wasn't until the mid-1960s that a successful chemotherapy protocol that produced long-term remissions was finally put into place – this used a range of drugs in combination and was used to treat children with ALL. Subsequent early successes included finding a combination protocol for both Hodgkin's and non-Hodgkin's lymphomas.

There are three important things to note from this story. The first is that some of these early drugs are still in clinical use – the nitrogen mustard agent became cyclophosphamide, the anti-folate became methotrexate, both drugs with widespread use in a range of different cancers even today. Secondly, the problem of resistance to therapy was apparent almost immediately – the short remissions were evidence that the tumours became resistant to the effects of these highly toxic and yet initially very successful drugs. Finally, and perhaps most importantly, all of these early successes were in haematological cancers – leukaemias and lymphomas – and not in the solid tumours such as breast, prostate, lung and the other major sites of disease.

In many respects these early successes in cancer chemotherapy set the stage for later developments – in particular two key principles were established. The first is that combination chemotherapy offers the best prospects for reducing the effects of induced resistance. The second is the use of very high-doses of these drugs to 'flood' the system in order to knock the disease out quickly. To this day this remains the basis for many of the protocols still used to treat cancers – including the solid tumours which actually make up the majority of cases of the disease [1].

## Maximum Tolerated Dose (MTD) Chemotherapy

The technical name for this standard treatment strategy is called maximum tolerated dose (MTD), or sometimes dose dense (DD), chemotherapy. The idea is very simple. There is a dose dependent effect of these highly toxic drugs on tumours – the more drug the greater the effect. When developing the protocols for using the drugs, the researchers have carried out a series of Phase I clinical trials which have established a maximum tolerated dose – this is the dose at which the majority of patients are able to cope with the side-effects, even when these are severe. Once this dose is established, then it can be used in the subsequent Phase II and Phase III trials which are more clearly looking for evidence that the drugs are effective against the disease itself (please read the chapters on clinical trials for more details).

The main reason for the side effects is that these drugs are delivered at high doses so that they can reach the cancer cells, which may be deep inside a tumour and not easily accessible to a chemical in the bloodstream. As the drugs circulate through the bloodstream they come into contact with cells throughout the body. Unfortunately most drugs are not able to distinguish between a 'good' cell and a 'bad' one – which means that the chemotherapy will also affect non-cancer cells. Some chemotherapy drugs target cells which are rapidly dividing – which is something that cancer cells do – but it also means that other rapidly dividing cells are also damaged. Examples include cells in the immune system, stomach lining and hair follicles. This is why some of the most common side effects of chemotherapy include immune suppression (neutropenia), nausea and vomiting and hair loss.

These side effects necessarily entail some recovery time for the patient – the immune system needs to recover, patients need to rest, the sickness has to subside. Commonly chemotherapy protocols are designed so that multiple chemotherapy drugs are combined and given over a set schedule which includes regular 'off-treatment' periods between cycles. Unfortunately, this recovery time can also be useful to the tumour – some cells which are resistant to the chemotherapy drug are able to recover and multiply in the time that the patient is also recovering. This leads to resistance to the chemotherapy as gradually the cells which are sensitive are removed by the chemo and those that remain and prosper are those most resistant. Such cells can often become 'multi-drug resistant', which means that their cellular machinery evolves to resist a wide range of different chemotherapy drugs.

287

It is not uncommon, therefore, to find that patients have very good initial responses to chemotherapy, with high rates of tumour regression, but that over time the response changes and the degree of tumour regression slows or even reverses and growth recommences. The tumours grow resistant to the treatment, and in some cases become more aggressive and resistant to other drugs too (a phenomenon termed multi-drug resistance).

## Low Dose Metronomic Chemotherapy

In contrast to MTD chemotherapy, the metronomic alternative does not include treatment breaks – there is no recovery time included in the protocols [2]. The reason for this is that the chemotherapy is prescribed at sufficiently low doses that the side effects do not kick in. Crucially, it has been shown that at these lower doses, these chemotherapy drugs, including the first generation drugs such as cyclophosphamide and methotrexate, work in radically different ways to how they work at higher doses. Whereas these drugs are very efficient cytotoxics (cell killing agents) at high doses, when used at low doses they do not directly kill cells, not even cancer cells. And by not killing cells the normal negative effects on non-cancer cells do not occur – there is no hair loss, vomiting or immune suppression as with normal chemotherapy.

This isn't to say that there are no side effects at all with metronomic chemotherapy – but these tend to be much less severe and debilitating than the side effects of high dose treatments. Some patients will develop low level fatigue, anaemia or diarrhoea for example. But these cases tend to be in the minority of patients treated metronomically and the severity of these symptoms is usually manageable. In contrast to standard dosing of chemotherapy, patients do not usually require dose reductions or treatment breaks.

However, despite not directly killing cancer cells there is strong evidence, including clinical trial evidence, that low dose metronomic chemotherapy does have a positive therapeutic effect. There have been numerous clinical trials which have reported positive results in terms of both long-term disease control rates and in some cases partial or complete regressions [3]. This naturally begs the question, if metronomic chemotherapy has lower toxicity and still shows good results, why isn't it used all the time? Before looking at how metronomic chemotherapy works it is important to look at the issues which surround this mode of treatment.

## Maintenance Protocols

Despite positive results in clinical trials and in numerous animal and laboratory studies, the area of oncology where metronomic chemotherapy is most often used is in patients who are in late stage disease. This is a population that has often been through numerous rounds of treatment, frequently including multiple lines of MTD chemotherapy. In the terminology of cancer this a patient population most often described as 'heavily pre-treated'. In practice this means not only that patients have got active, often aggressive, cancers, but that they are also carrying the after-effects of those rounds of maximum dose chemotherapy, radiotherapy, surgery and more. At this stage most oncologists are no longer looking for disease remissions but are thinking in terms of maintenance therapies to keep the disease at bay for as long as possible.

This is the context in which patients are more likely to be offered a metronomic chemotherapy protocol. It is also the case that the majority of clinical trials of metronomic chemotherapy have been in this patient population – which makes the positive results which have been reported quite remarkable at times, particularly the small number of cases of disease regression rather than just the stable disease that is what is hoped for. In contrast, trials of maximum dose chemotherapy, in the same population, generally do not yield many regressions or even disease control.

Given these results, it is even more surprising that even in this heavily pre-treated population more patients are *not* offered the chance to go on metronomic protocols rather than trying yet another high-dose chemotherapy regimen. Unfortunately it is the case that many oncologists do not actively consider metronomic protocols even in late stage patients and, in some cases, are highly resistant to the idea even when it has been suggested to them directly by patients, patient advocates or other clinicians.

## Mechanisms of Action

As previously mentioned it is known that when used at low doses many of these highly toxic chemotherapy drugs no longer work as cytotoxic agents. Instead it is now known that there are two main mechanisms of action which explain the therapeutic effects.

### Angiogenesis

The first mechanism of action is related to angiogenesis. This term describes the sprouting of new blood vessels and is a natural process which normally occurs in wound healing. The new blood vessels sprout from the existing vessels, creating a new network that can supply oxygen and nutrients from the bloodstream to the tissues that need it for wound repair. However, this process is also used by tumours and it is considered one of the six 'hallmarks of cancer' [4].

Tumours are rapidly growing collections of cells, with a need for oxygen and nutrients from the blood supply in order to survive and expand. Without this blood supply the tumour cells will be starved of oxygen and nutrients and will eventually die. But, unfortunately, cancers are able to switch on the process that triggers the formation of new blood vessels. As the tumours expand, they can keep it switched on, so that there is an ever expanding network of blood vessels, to keep the rapidly expanding tumour mass supplied with the fuels and raw materials it needs for continued and accelerating growth.

This process is properly termed tumour neo-angiogenesis and is the subject of a huge research effort, both to understand the details of how it occurs and also to find ways of shutting it off. A number of drugs have been developed which aim to switch off the process of angiogenesis – this class of agents are called anti-angiogenic drugs or angiogenesis inhibitors, and the most famous of these is the drug bevacizumab (more commonly known by its trade name of Avastin). Drugs like bevacizumab target specific chemical signals that are assumed to be key to that process. The angiogenic process is controlled by a series of different chemical signals which

- initiate the budding of new vessels from old
- signal for the new buds to expand and extend
- finally other signals kick in which are meant to end the process.

These chemical signals are released by cells from the immune system, from cells called fibroblasts and other cells which surround the tumour (collectively these cells are termed the tumour microenvironment). Furthermore the tumours themselves release factors which mean that the shut-off signals are blocked, and release other chemical signals which drive the process forward still further.

The idea behind anti-angiogenic therapy therefore is simple – if we can stop the sprouting of new blood vessels, then the tumour will not be able to sustain its high growth rate – it will literally be starved of nutrients and not be able to continue to expand. At the very least it is hoped that this will stop tumour growth in its tracks, and, eventually, lead to tumour shrinkage as existing cancer cells die.

Coming back to metronomics, it is now known that at low doses many chemotherapy drugs act on the angiogenic process [5]. They can in fact block or even reverse the process of angiogenesis. They do this *not* by blocking specific chemical signals in the way that bevacizumab or other 'targeted angiogenesis inhibitors' do, but by acting on the *cells* which release those signals. In other words metronomic chemotherapy does not act on very specific chemical signals but on the cells which release or process those signals. These are the cells of the tumour microenvironment – particularly fibroblasts and tumour-associated endothelial cells. This is an important difference for two reasons.

The first is that there are many different chemical pathways involved in angiogenesis, blocking one specific signal with a drug like bevacizumab does not mean that the process ends. There are often alternative signals which kick in and after an initial reduction in angiogenesis the process picks up again. This manifests itself when drugs like bevacizumab stop working in patients – acquired resistance to targeted angiogenesis drugs is frequent and well-known. In contrast, acting on the tumour microenvironment – the cells of which release many of these signals – may be more effective because it blocks *multiple* signals at the same time. It also acts on some of the cells which process these signals, again acting to reduce angiogenesis.

Secondly, cancer cells have very high mutation rates – this is one of the things that makes cancer cells different to non-cancer cells. This means that cells in the tumour can adapt and change in response to treatment – this is what drives the emergence of resistance to therapies. In the case of angiogenesis it means that cancer cells which produce a particular chemical signal that is blocked by a drug such as bevacizumab may develop a mutation that overrides the action of that drug. Those cells with this mutation will therefore survive and out-compete the sensitive cells so that, in time, the population of resistant cells expands and the tumour continues to grow. In contrast the cells in the tumour microenvironment, which are not cancerous and have much lower mutation rates, are less likely to develop resistance.

The upshot of this is that, by acting on the microenvironment, low-dose metronomic chemotherapy can have a broader and more sustained anti-angiogenic action than some of the more expensive and more toxic drugs which are specifically targeted at the chemical signals controlling angiogenesis. In practice, this means that metronomic chemotherapy can be very effective in cutting off the growing blood supply that feeds tumours. Effectively it means that tumours stop expanding aggressively, and in some cases they may even begin to shrink slowly.

## Immune Response

The second main mechanism of action is immune-related. Where standard chemotherapy often leads to immune suppression and the emergence of populations of immune cells which are actually pro-tumour, metronomic chemotherapy can have a positive effect on anticancer immunity.

In the past it was assumed that cancer was invisible to the immune system, but we now know that the reality is far more complex than that. There are in fact populations of immune cells which can act either for or against cancer. Cells such as macrophages, neutrophils and platelets can switch from being anticancer to pro-cancer. We know there are populations of cells called myeloid derived suppressor cells (MDSCs) and T-regulatory cells (T-reg) cells, which are actively involved in subverting the immune response to cancer. And, as with angiogenesis, tumours release chemical signals which can encourage these pro-cancer immune populations and discourage the activity of the anticancer immune cells.

In contrast to high-dose chemotherapy, there is strong evidence that some chemotherapy drugs have activity against these populations of pro-cancer immune cells when used at metronomic doses [6]. By acting in this way these drugs can interrupt the subversion of the immune system and therefore allow the anticancer immune cells to act against the tumour.

## Other Mechanisms

As with other topics in cancer our understanding of metronomic chemotherapy is still expanding through laboratory studies in addition to clinical experience. An emerging theme in our understanding of metronomic chemotherapy is the role that it has in influencing tumour evolution. Cancers are composed of mixed populations of cancer cells, in competition with each other and with non-cancer cells. As cells divide they mutate, the daughter cells grow and divide and some of them will mutate in turn. This leads to sub-populations of cells in a tumour having different genetic make-up. Some of them may be more sensitive to chemotherapy and some less. When we use standard high-dose chemotherapy we effectively inflict massive tumour kill by wiping out the most sensitive cells. But the cells that survive will be more resistant and will now have less competition for resources from the sensitive cells that have been killed. Over time these resistant cells will further mutate and expand, so that successive chemotherapy treatments have the effect of weeding out the most sensitive and least aggressive cells. In time the remaining cells often become 'multi-drug' resistant.

However, because metronomic chemotherapy is not directly targeting the cancer cells this weeding out of sensitive cells does not occur. The mixed population of sensitive and resistant cells remains in place. This keeps the competition for resources in place, and does not give the advantage to the more aggressive and resistant cancers to emerge as the dominant population. There is now an interest in combining metronomic chemotherapy with standard high-dose chemotherapy in so-called 'chemo-switch' protocols. In one scenario the high-dose chemotherapy is not used frequently but is added in as an occasional treatment to take advantage of the massive tumour kill alongside the metronomic chemotherapy. Because the high-dose chemo is not used successively the weeding out of all the more sensitive cells does not take place to the same extent.

## Resistance to Metronomic Chemotherapy

While there are numerous positive aspects to metronomic chemotherapy there remains much that we do not understand about it. A particular problem is that despite long-term disease stabilisation in many patients – in some cases extending to years – for many patients resistance eventually emerges even with this treatment. It is widely believed that the mechanism of resistance is different to the resistance to maximum tolerated dose chemotherapy. Evidence for this comes from the fact that mouse tumours that have become resistant to low dose metronomic cyclophosphamide are still sensitive to high-doses of the drug and vice versa. It is also clear that resistance to one drug at metronomic doses does not equate to resistance to all drugs at metronomic doses – in contrast to the situation of multi-drug resistance in high-dose chemotherapy.

However, there is intense on-going research to develop new protocols that improve response and limit the emergence of resistance. As with combination therapies in standard treatment, it is clear that the best results are likely to arise from combination protocols with metronomic chemotherapy. Common protocols which are currently in clinical trial include:

- Combinations of metronomic chemotherapy agents. For example daily oral cyclophosphamide and capecitabine, methotrexate or other low dose chemotherapy drug.

- Combinations of metronomic chemotherapy with high-dose chemotherapy. For example metronomic chemotherapy in combination with high dose cisplatin or doxorubicin.
- Metronomic chemotherapy with a targeted therapy. For example low dose cyclophosphamide with bevacizumab.
- Metronomic chemotherapy in combination with non-cytotoxic drugs, for example the anti-inflammatory pain-killer celecoxib.

One area that is just starting to be explored in clinical trials, but which has been actively researched in laboratory studies, involves the use of metronomic chemotherapy in combination with non-cancer drugs. Examples include the anti-diabetic drug metformin, the beta-blocker propranolol, the anti-cholesterol statin drugs, the anti-epileptic drug valproic acid and many more. These are examples of drug repurposing, a topic we will come to in the next chapter.

Tumour dormancy may also be a long-term issue with metronomic chemotherapy. Given that the treatment itself does not directly kill cancer cells, it is possible for small pockets of malignant cells to enter a dormant state in which they effectively go into a 'sleep mode' for the duration of the treatment.

These dormant cells may not show up on scans and present no immediate medical problem, as the metronomic treatment keeps them shut down. However, when the metronomic treatment ends, perhaps after many months without apparent sign of disease, the cells can once again 'wake up' and become active.

While there is much active research into these issues – there are currently well over 100 trials of metronomic chemotherapy listed in the various clinical trial registries – for the moment these issues have to be taken seriously. However, when there are no other alternatives, and certainly no other alternatives with the same low toxicity, then metronomic chemotherapy can be an attractive proposition, at least for late-stage cancer patients.

There is even an argument to be made that we have our current treatment priorities wrong – that perhaps it is better to *start* with the low dose metronomic chemotherapy early in the disease process and to switch to the higher dose therapies later on. Early-stage disease imposes a lower burden on the patient and is possibly more likely to benefit from the disease stabilisation that metronomics can provide. Perhaps we should switch to the higher toxicity treatments only when the disease has started to progress in the face of resistance to metronomic chemotherapy. Another appealing approach is to use a 'chemo-switch' approach which uses a mixture of high-dose and metronomic dose treatments [7]. However, this is the personal view of the author and it is unlikely that the change in practice that this would entail will happen until there are some major Phase III trial results to prove once and for all the efficacy of such treatments.

## Searching For Metronomic Options

The starting point for anyone looking for metronomic options is a clinical trials registry such as clinicatrials.gov or the UK clinical trials gateway (http://www.ukctg.nihr.ac.uk/default.aspx). For more details on these and other options for finding clinical trials please refer to the chapter entitled 'Accessing Clinical Trials'.

To get the best results use queries that include the type of cancer with an appropriate keyword, for example 'metronomic' or 'low dose chemotherapy'. For example on clinicaltrials.gov the simple search 'breast cancer metronomic' returns 22 open trials.

Summary

- Standard chemotherapy, also known as 'maximum tolerated dose' (MTD) chemotherapy, works on the principle of applying combinations of high-dose toxic chemotherapy with the aim of maximising tumour reduction
- Treatment breaks are required in MTD chemotherapy protocols so that patients can recover from the side effects of the drugs
- Low-dose metronomic chemotherapy is an alternative approach that uses low doses of standard chemotherapy such that they do not cause significant side effects. This means that the drugs can be administered continuously and without treatment breaks
- Metronomic chemotherapy does not aim to directly cause massive tumour kill but instead it attacks the tumour blood supply by acting on the tumour microenvironment – depriving tumours of the blood and oxygen they need to continue to grow
- In contrast to MTD chemotherapy the metronomic protocols do not cause suppression of the immune system and in some cases actually attack the population of immune cells which support the tumour
- There are encouraging results in many cancer types using a range of different chemotherapy drugs in metronomic mode
- There is much on-going research, including many clinical trials in different cancer types

and in combination with many different drugs

- While stable disease can often be achieved, and in some cases significant partial or full regression, resistance to treatment can still occur

## References

1 Crawford S (2013) **Is it time for a new paradigm for systemic cancer treatment? Lessons from a century of cancer chemotherapy.** *Frontiers in pharmacology*, **4**(June), p. 68.

2 Scharovsky OG, Mainetti LE and Rozados VR (2009) **Metronomic chemotherapy: changing the paradigm that more is better.** *Current oncology (Toronto, Ont.)*, **16**(2), pp. 7–15.

3 Montagna E, Cancello G, Dellapasqua S, Munzone E and Colleoni M (2014) **Metronomic therapy and breast cancer: a systematic review.** *Cancer treatment reviews*, **40**(8), pp. 942–50.

4 Hanahan D and Weinberg RA (2011) **Hallmarks of cancer: the next generation.** *Cell*, **144**(5), pp. 646–74.

5     Drevs J, Fakler J, Eisele S, Medinger M, et al. (2004) **Antiangiogenic potency of various chemotherapeutic drugs for metronomic chemotherapy.** *Anticancer research*, **24**(3a), pp. 1759–63.

6     Kareva I, Waxman DJ and Klement GL (2014) **Metronomic chemotherapy: An attractive alternative to maximum tolerated dose therapy that can activate anti-tumor immunity and minimize therapeutic resistance.** *Cancer letters*, **358**(2), pp. 14–17.

7     Malik PS, Raina V and André N (2014) **Metronomics as maintenance treatment in oncology: time for chemo-switch.** *Frontiers in oncology*, **4**(April), p. 76.

# Drug Repurposing

## Introduction

Before looking at the main topic of this chapter –
drug repurposing – it is worth digressing briefly to
look at how new cancer drugs are generally
developed. In recent years the dominant trend in
cancer drug development has been to focus on a
class of drugs called 'targeted therapies'. Where
many chemotherapy drugs aim to kill rapidly
dividing cells – which means that both cancer and
non-cancer cells are affected – targeted therapies are
aimed instead at very specific molecular targets (i.e.
they are based on very specific mechanisms at work
inside cancer cells). Based on our increasing
understanding of cancer at the detailed molecular
level, these drugs seek to inhibit tumour growth by
disrupting specific cellular pathways and networks.
If we think of cells as little boxes of biological
circuitry then targeted therapies aim to interfere with
bits of the circuit inside the box in order to stop it
working properly, in contrast, old-fashioned
chemotherapy tried to blow the whole box up.

As will be outlined later, there are some significant
issues with some of these targeted therapies, as well
as some significant successes. However, the targeted

approach is not the only one, and one alternative approach is called drug repurposing. In this approach the existing supply of non-cancer medicines is viewed as a potential source of new drugs which have some value in cancer treatments. This chapter will explore some of the ideas behind these different approaches to cancer drug discovery and also highlight a number of drugs which have been identified to date as having some potential. In addition please refer to the chapter on Metronomic Chemotherapy for a discussion on another alternative to high-dose chemotherapy.

## Targeted Therapies

The promise of targeted agents is that they are aimed very precisely at specific pathways (biological circuits) that cancers use to survive and thrive. In contrast to the scatter-gun approach of standard high-dose chemotherapy, these drugs are molecularly targeted so that they interfere with processes that are essential for tumour survival. Very often this means not killing cancer cells directly but rather tackling some of the support systems that tumours depend on.

For example tumours need oxygen and nutrients in order to grow, just like other cells in the body, so a process called angiogenesis kicks in (this was also discussed in the chapter on metronomic chemotherapy). Angiogenesis is a natural process that is used by the body in wound healing; it ensures that small vessels sprout from existing ones and that blood can flow into the areas that are needed to heal cuts. But when tumours exploit angiogenesis they use it to make sure they can get the blood and oxygen they need to expand – and as the tumour expands so does the blood supply. Interrupting this process would put a brake on that tumour growth – and so targeted drugs have been developed which specifically interfere with the chemical signals and processes that tumours use to control angiogenesis.

Another main area of development of targeted therapies is immunotherapy. Tumours evolve so that they disarm or subvert the response of the immune system, which would otherwise attack them. For example, they release chemical signals to attract some types of immune cells that protect the tumour from populations of anti-tumour immune cells. Therefore a new generation of targeted agents has been developed which interfere with this subversion process so that the immune system can kick in and destroy the tumours.

However, while these targeted therapies can produce some fantastic responses initially, there are also some fairly major issues associated with them. The first and most important is that very often the impressive responses are temporary. This is because the body contains multiple redundant circuits – there are many different pathways involved in angiogenesis for example – and so when one pathway is blocked another pathway may become active (think of cutting off the power to a computer only to find that there's a backup power supply that can kick in and keep it working). Tumours are evolutionary systems that contain different populations of cells, and while the vast majority may depend on the pathway that is blocked it only needs one cell that uses an alternative pathway for resistance to emerge later. Over time, the cells which are sensitive to the drug will die, but in their place the cells which are resistant will expand in numbers and become the dominant cell population in the tumour.

A second issue with targeted agents is that frequently these drugs are also highly toxic. Many targeted agents have significant side effects associated with them – and these may mean that patients have to come off the treatment.

Finally, it also needs pointing out that many of these new targeted agents are hugely expensive – which imposes financial burdens on the NHS and may mean that supplies of these drugs are rationed or even that NICE (National Institute of Clinical Excellence, the body that decides which drugs can be used in the NHS), refuses to make the drugs available at all.


## Repurposing As a Strategy

Drug repurposing is not a new idea, in fact there are numerous examples where a drug that has been developed for one disease is subsequently found to be active in another. Possibly the most famous example is viagra, which was initially developed as an anti-angina drug for patients with heart disease. However, it turned out that the drug was very effective as a treatment for erectile dysfunction – for which it is now primarily used. In terms of cancer, the story has not been so positive. There are a number of cancer drugs which have since been reused in non-cancer diseases – for example one of the first cancer drugs was methotrexate, which is still used to treat osteosarcoma and other cancers, but which is now also being used to treat rheumatoid arthritis. Another example is the targeted anti-cancer agent bevacizumab (Avastin), which was developed as an anti-angiogenic drug for cancer but is now also being used to treat macular degeneration.

What about non-cancer drugs being used in cancer? The picture there is not so rosy. To date the only non-cancer drug in regular clinical use as a cancer treatment is the drug thalidomide. This was originally used to treat morning sickness in pregnancy, but was soon found to cause severe birth defects. However, the drug is now a standard anti-angiogenic treatment that is used primarily in multiple myeloma.

This is not to say that there are no other drugs with the potential to be used in cancer treatments. Currently there is a huge degree of interest in a number of very common drugs, particularly aspirin, the anti-diabetic drug metformin and in some statins. The Repurposing Drugs in Oncology (ReDO) project, of which this author is a member, is a scientific project that is actively investigating a number of less common non-cancer drugs which also have some potential as cancer treatments [1,2]. Before moving on to look at particular repurposed drugs we should perhaps touch briefly on some of the advantages that the repurposing approach promises.

One immediate and obvious benefit is that by using well-known drugs with many years of clinical use we can take advantage of all the data that is available on side-effects, (including rare side effects that only emerge after a drug has been used for many years), dosing and treatment schedules. In contrast when we are dealing with new drugs there is scant data available and in many cases numerous rounds of clinical trials are required to identify the best doses, likely side effects and treatment schedules. Aside from the patient safety angle, this is important because it can potentially short-circuit the drug development process. While it can take many years before a new drug can actually reach the point where it can be tested for effectiveness (see the two chapters on clinical trials for more details), there is the potential for repurposed drugs to skip the early phase trials and go direct to Phase II or Phase III trials.

Related to the safety angle is a positive toxicity profile. These drugs often do not cause the kinds of problems that many chemotherapy or targeted therapy drugs do. Although this does not mean that there are no side-effects to treatment, these are often easily manageable and do not impose negative impacts on the quality of life of the patients taking these drugs.

Another distinct advantage derives from the fact that many of these drugs are off-patent (i.e. they are no longer protected by patent law and can be manufactured by many different companies without having to pay expensive licence fees) and available as generics (unbranded – a bit like a supermarket 'own-brand' product compared to a brand-name product). This means the drugs are often very cheap and easily sourced. In contrast, the newest generation of targeted drugs have a very high price tags attached – it is not uncommon for these drugs to cost tens of thousands per treatment cycle. While these prices are not paid directly by patients in the NHS, it does impose a significant financial burden that can lead to drug rationing or even a refusal by NICE to allow the supply of a drug altogether.

It should be noted that it's important that we keep in mind that the key criterion for assessing these drugs is not toxicity or cost, it's that they display evidence of anti-cancer activity at clinically relevant doses. This means looking for evidence of effect using data from clinical trials and case reports, not just depending on laboratory data in animals or test tubes. In other words, even though these are existing drugs that are widely used, they still have to go through the clinical trials process to confirm whether or not they have a beneficial effect when added to cancer treatments.

The end-point of drug repurposing research is to get these old drugs 're-licensed' for use as cancer treatments, once the benefit is confirmed in clinical trials, and to have them adopted as 'standard of care'. This means that these drugs become part of normal medical practice and are included as part of the standard treatment protocols for different cancers. Doctors, in the UK and many other countries, are able to prescribe any licensed drug to their patients if they believe the drug will be beneficial. This mean a doctor is able to prescribe a drug 'off-label', in other words a doctor is able to prescribe a drug for an illness for which the drug is not licensed – so in theory a doctor is able to prescribe one of these repurposed drugs before it has been re-licensed. However, this is not a preferred long-term solution, which is to make those repurposed drugs part of standard practice and licensed for new uses in cancer treatment.

## Repurposed Drugs

The following is a selection of the many drugs which have some evidence of clinical activity that is relevant in a cancer setting. At the moment none of them is in use as part of standard of care therapy, although many of them are being investigated in clinical trials and in some cases there are clinicians who are prescribing these drugs to their patients as 'off-label' therapies.

## Aspirin

While aspirin has a recognised role in the prevention of heart disease, there is increasing recognition that it also has a role both in the prevention and treatment of cancer [3]. In terms of cancer prevention there is evidence from numerous epidemiological studies (i.e. studies of large populations) that it can help reduce the incidence of the disease in a range of different cancer types, including colorectal, oesophageal, biliary and breast cancer. The effect is apparent for long-term users – that is people who have been using aspirin for longer than 3 years – and appears to apply to low-dose aspirin (75 mg/day) as well as higher doses (300 mg/day). There are some indications that this long term effect may be due to aspirin reducing the chance that primary tumours metastasise (spread) to distant organs.

While the major emphasis in research has been on looking at aspirin for cancer prevention in high risk groups – such as those suffering from Lynch Syndrome (a genetic cancer predisposition syndrome) – there is now also an interest in using aspirin as a cancer treatment. Currently there is evidence in colorectal and breast cancer that taking aspirin post-diagnosis has a positive effect on disease free survival and overall survival [4,5]. There is also some evidence – though not as strong – that aspirin can improve survival following surgical resection in non-small cell lung cancer [6].

The evidence for a positive effect of aspirin as a cancer treatment is sufficiently strong that there is now a large Phase III randomised trial in the UK and India which will assess the impact of aspirin on four different cancers: breast, colorectal, oesophageal and prostate. This large trial will recruit 11,000 patients in total. Some will be randomised to receive a dummy tablet, some will receive a low dose (100 mg) tablet and some a high dose tablet (300 mg). All groups will take one tablet a day for five years.

It should be noted that the effect is likely to be greater for those suffering from early stage disease, particularly for those who do not have metastatic disease. There is currently little evidence that aspirin has an effect on late-stage disease.

There are of course risks with every drug, and that includes aspirin. Daily aspirin can increase the risk of gastrointestinal bleeding, and should be avoided by those at high risk of bleeds, for example those with existing stomach ulcers. The risks of bleeding can be reduced if aspirin is taken with food or with a proton pump inhibitor (e.g. omeprazole, lansoprazole etc) or other antacid.

## Metformin

Most commonly prescribed as a routine part of the treatment for type II diabetes, metformin is another drug which is attracting a good degree of attention as a potential additional treatment for cancer [7,8]. As with aspirin the initial evidence for an effect came from epidemiological studies that showed that diabetes patients on metformin had lower incidence of cancer compared to diabetics on other medication. This was followed up with laboratory and animal studies that showed that metformin had a number of different effects on cancer cells.

While metformin is not yet in common use in oncology, there is a very significant level of clinical trial activity. Currently there are clinical trials in a very wide range of cancers, including cancers of the breast, prostate, lung, brain and skin cancers. These trials cover both early stage and advanced disease, included metastatic cancers. There are also trials that cover paediatric cancers as well as in adults. Currently, in June 2015, there are over 80 trials in metformin listed as recruiting or about to start recruiting. However, to date there have been very few results reported from randomised clinical trials – but the first of these, in pancreatic cancer, failed to show any benefit from the addition of metformin.

It is also the case that some patients are treated with metformin outside of a formal clinical trial. The evidence is sufficiently convincing that some oncologists prescribe metformin 'off-label' for their patients, particularly in the case of patients who have been through first or second-line treatment and still have active disease. In some cases patients have also been advised by oncologists to approach their GPs to get a prescription for metformin. However, the recommended starting point for a patient wishing to explore the addition of metformin to their treatment should be a search for an appropriate clinical trial.

### Itraconazole

While aspirin and metformin are both being very actively pursued by the medical research community, the same cannot be said for itraconazole. This is a standard anti-fungal treatment that is used to treat a range of conditions caused by fungal infections, including candida infections (thrush). It does have use in cancer treatment, but only as an anti-fungal agent used to prevent such infections in high-risk patients. It is also used for long term prevention of fungal infection in patients with depressed immunity, such as HIV patients. As such this is a drug that can be used safely for extended periods and with minimal side effects.

Laboratory evidence has shown that itraconazole has a number of anticancer properties that make it a potentially useful addition to treatment [9]. It has been shown to reverse drug resistance in some types of cancer cells which are resistant to chemotherapy. Additionally there is evidence that it works as an anti-angiogenic agent, thereby reducing the growth of the pro-tumour blood supply that is an essential part of the cancer growth process. And finally there is some evidence that it blocks a specific signalling pathway called the Hedgehog pathway – one of the biological circuits of interest to those developing new targeted therapies.

In terms of clinical evidence there have been a small number of clinical trials which have looked specifically at the anticancer effect of itraconazole. The best evidence to date is in castration-resistant metastatic prostate cancer, non-small cell lung cancer and in basal cell carcinoma. These are also the cancers in which there are clinical trials currently on-going. It is to be hoped that additional trials will be initiated in the near future. Certainly the evidence in these cancers is strongest, but there is also some evidence that itraconazole may be effective in breast cancer, glioblastoma, ovarian cancer and pancreatic cancer.

## Cimetidine

Cimetidine (also known by the trade name Tagamet) is another old drug which has considerable levels of evidence to suggest it is of some benefit to cancer patients [10,11]. Cimetidine is an antacid that has been in common use for decades – though increasingly it is being replaced by newer drugs such as the proton pump inhibitors (omeprazole, pantoprazole etc). In some countries cimetidine is available as an over the counter drug, in others it remains a prescription only medicine.

Unlike itraconazole there is ample clinical evidence of an anticancer effect of cimetidine in people, in addition to numerous laboratory studies which explain the different mechanisms of action. The main mechanisms of action are via effects on tumour cell proliferation (the rate of growth of tumour cells), on angiogenesis and, possibly the most significant, positive effects on the immune system. There are multiple different effects on immunity, but the most significant are in terms of reversing the immune suppression induced by tumour growth, thereby allowing immune cells to more easily penetrate and attack tumours.

While there is some evidence in humans for a range of cancers, including melanoma, gastric cancer and renal cell carcinoma, it is in colorectal cancer that we have the most evidence. There have been a number of different trials in colorectal cancer which have shown a positive effect of cimetidine when it is administered alongside surgical resection of the tumour. These trials were performed in different countries and at different times, so it is difficult to draw firm conclusions about the best dose and schedule to use. A Cochrane Review (which applies the strictest criteria to evaluate data from multiple studies) concluded that perioperative cimetidine is associated with reduced immunosuppression and a lower risk of disease recurrence in the curative resection of colorectal cancer [12]. It is extremely disappointing that these positive results have not been translated into changes in clinical practice. However, there is a large trial of cimetidine in colorectal cancer underway in Australia and New Zealand which will hopefully confirm previous results and lead to the adoption of cimetidine as a standard part of colorectal cancer treatment.

Colorectal cancer is not the only form of the disease which might benefit from cimetidine, the mechanisms of action are not specific to cells in the colon but would, in theory, apply to all cancers. It should also be noted that these effects seem to be specific to cimetidine and do not seem to apply to some of the other drugs in the same class, such as loratidine, which is available over the counter.

## Mebendazole

Mebendazole is a common anti-parasitic drug used to treat helminths infections – this includes threadworms, tapeworms and roundworms – in both humans and animals. It is available over the counter and has a very good safety and toxicity profile. It also has some evidence that it is another multi-targeted anticancer agent with good potential for being repurposed [13]. The evidence comes largely from laboratory experiments and some case reports, but the data is sufficiently interesting that a small number of clinical trials are currently underway, primarily in glioblastoma. However, the evidence suggests that mebendazole should be of value in other cancers, particularly in melanoma, non-small cell lung cancer, colorectal cancer and possibly also in breast cancer and osteosarcoma.

There are multiple mechanisms of action at work. The first is that it acts as a microtubule disrupter, which is what the more toxic drugs in the taxane class (taxol and docetaxel) and the vinca alkaloids (vincristine and vinblastine) also do. Microtubule disruption effectively interferes with the process of cells dividing and so this can slow or stop tumour growth. Additionally there is some evidence that mebendazole is anti-angiogenic and can also, like itraconazole, target the Hedgehog signalling pathway.

It is to be hoped that if the small on-going clinical trials on-going report positive results then mebendazole can be added to clinical practice and also that it is investigated in a wider range of cancer types.

## Clarithromycin

So far we have looked at an anti-fungal drug and an anti-parasitic, this begs the question of whether we shouldn't also look at antibiotics as a source of anticancer drugs. In fact there are a range of antibiotics which do show some evidence of activity, including clarithromycin, doxycycline and minocycline. We should also point out that some standard chemotherapy drugs, such as doxorubicin (also called adriamycin) belong to a class of drugs called anti-tumour antibiotics. These drugs are extremely toxic and are not used as antibiotics to treat infections, they are used instead in cancer treatments for their anti-tumour effect. In contrast clarithromycin and doxycycline are both standard antibiotics used to treat a broad spectrum of common bacterial infections.

Clarithromycin has solid clinical evidence primarily in two cancers, multiple myeloma and the rare lymphoma Waldenström's macroglobulinemia [14]. Positive results have also been reported in other haematological cancers, particularly when clarithromycin is used with dexamethasone and other agents. Clinical trials are clearly warranted in these cancers in order to prove efficacy and initiate the process of changing practice. The evidence is less clear in solid tumours, although there are indications from small clinical trials that clarithromycin has a positive effect in non-small cell lung cancer. Given that clarithromycin is a cheap drug, available as a generic, and has low toxicity associated with it clinical trials are urgently needed to move things forward.

## Nitroglycerin

Nitroglycerin, also known as glyceryl trinitrate, is another drug with a long history of clinical use – in this case it's one of the oldest and most established drugs for the treatment of angina. It belongs to a type of drug called a vasodilator, which means that it relaxes or widens the blood vessels, causing a lowering of blood pressure. It's a very fast-acting drug, most often administered as a spray under the tongue or via transdermal patches worn on the skin. There is now an interest in exploiting these clinical effects for anti-cancer purposes [15]. Focus on the anticancer activity of nitroglycerin is directed at two specific mechanisms.

The first is to do with the effect on the blood vessels. As has been mentioned, tumours are very good at kicking off the process of angiogenesis so that they can recruit a local blood supply. This blood supply is frequently chaotic and leaky compared to normal blood vessels. By taking nitroglycerin at the same time as chemotherapy the leaky vessels can be widened in order to accentuate the leakiness. This causes the chemotherapy drugs to leak out from the blood vessels and into the tumour tissue, where they can have more of an effect. This is called the enhanced permeability and retention effect, and there is much research on selecting the right combination of drugs to achieve a better targeting of drugs to the tumours .

Additionally nitroglycerin has been used to improve response to radiotherapy. Again this is related to its effect on the blood vessels – in this case improved blood flow causes more oxygen supply into the tumour, which has the effect of improving the tumour kill caused by radiotherapy. The cancer in which there has been most work is lung cancer, and there are continuing clinical trials in Europe and other parts of the world exploring the combination of standard chemo-radiotherapy with the addition of nitroglycerin patches.

There is also interest in another facet of nitroglycerin, which is that it appears to have some effect on hypoxic tissues. Hypoxia means lack of oxygen and this is a problem associated with solid tumours. Hypoxia causes tumours to become more aggressive, to resist chemo and radiotherapy and to ultimately become more metastatic. Nitroglycerin has shown some evidence of reversing this hypoxia, including in clinical trials, both in lung cancer and in castration-resistant prostate cancer.

## Propranolol

Propranolol is another example of an old drug that is now exciting cancer researchers with its potential to make a clinical difference in cancer. It belongs to a class of drugs called beta blockers, which are used to treat high blood pressure as well as a range of other conditions. As with aspirin and metformin, there is solid epidemiological evidence for a positive effect of propranolol in some cancers, mainly through reducing the risk of metastatic spread [16].

There are multiple mechanisms thought to be involved in the anticancer effects of propranolol many of them involving beta-adrenergic signalling – this is the beta that beta-blockers stop – which is a key pathway involved in physical and psychological stress responses. This is especially active in the process by which metastatic tumours spread, particularly in the period following surgery. There is a huge level of interest therefore in tackling this post-surgical surge in metastatic spread [17]. There is evidence that propranolol, alone or in combination with drugs like etodolac (a drug similar to ketorolac and diclofenac), can have a positive impact in reducing post-surgical metastases in animal models [18].

However, there is also some very interesting and exciting data that shows that propranolol can have an impact on a rare cancer called angiosarcoma. This is a disease with no standard treatment, but doctors have successfully treated patients with the combination of metronomic chemotherapy and propranolol and have seen truly impressive results [19]. This work is now being extended into clinical trials in angiosarcoma and, hopefully, if the results are positive, this will lead to propranolol becoming the standard of care for this cancer. The hope is, of course, that the effect may also apply to other cancer types.

### Statins

Finally, mention should be made of another class of drug which is attracting a good deal of research interest from the oncology community and that is statins – which are prescribed to lower cholesterol with the intention of reducing the risk of heart attack [20]. There is a complex history around the link between cholesterol, saturated fats and heart disease but this is not the place to review this topic. Instead statins are attracting attention for similar reasons that aspirin and metformin did initially – that is there is evidence, from population studies, that statin use is associated with better outcomes in those cancer patients prescribed statins for heart disease than in cancer patients not on statins. This epidemiological evidence is also supported by laboratory studies in test tubes and in animals which show an anticancer effect. However, as with metformin, while there are many clinical trials on –going, or at a late stage of planning, to date there have been few convincing clinical trials delivering results one way or another.

## Summary

- Drug repurposing aims to take existing non-cancer drugs and re-use them in addition to other drugs as part of cancer treatment
- Many of the drugs of interest in repurposing are common drugs, often available as generics, with both low cost and low toxicity
- Some of the drugs of interest include: aspirin, metformin, itraconazole, mebendazole,

cimetidine, clarithromycin, nitroglycerin and statins

- While none of these drugs is part of standard cancer therapy, there are clinical trials in all of them and for any doctor or patient interested in exploring these drugs as a treatment option searching for a suitable clinical trial is recommended as a first step
- Some clinicians are willing to prescribe repurposed drugs in an 'off-label' way in certain cases

## References

1    Pantziarka P, Bouche G, Meheus L, Sukhatme V and Sukhatme VP (2014) **The Repurposing Drugs in Oncology (ReDO) Project.** *Ecancermedicalscience*, **8**, p. 442.

2    Pantziarka P, Bouche G, Meheus L, Sukhatme V and Sukhatme VP (2015) **Repurposing drugs in your medicine cabinet: untapped opportunities for cancer therapy?** *Future oncology (London, England)*, **11**(2), pp. 181–4.

3    Langley RE (2013) **Clinical evidence for the use of aspirin in the treatment of cancer.** *Ecancermedicalscience*, **7**(1), p. 297.

4       McCowan C, Munro  a J, Donnan PT and
        Steele RJC (2013) **Use of aspirin post-
        diagnosis in a cohort of patients with
        colorectal cancer and its association with
        all-cause and colorectal cancer specific
        mortality.** *European journal of cancer
        (Oxford, England : 1990)*, **49**(5), pp. 1049–57.

5       Fraser DM, Sullivan FM, Thompson  a M and
        McCowan C (2014) **Aspirin use and survival
        after the diagnosis of breast cancer: a
        population-based cohort study.** *British
        journal of cancer*, (April), pp. 1–5.

6       Wang H, Liao Z, Zhuang Y, Liu Y, et al.
        (2015) **Incidental receipt of cardiac
        medications and survival outcomes among
        patients with stage III non-small-cell lung
        cancer after definitive radiotherapy.**
        *Clinical lung cancer*, **16**(2), pp. 128–36.

7       Goodwin PJ, Ligibel JA and Stambolic V
        (2009) **Metformin in breast cancer: time for
        action.** *Journal of clinical oncology : official
        journal of the American Society of Clinical
        Oncology*, **27**(20), pp. 3271–3.

8       Dowling RJO, Niraula S, Stambolic V and
        Goodwin PJ (2012) **Metformin in cancer:
        translational challenges.** *Journal of*

*molecular endocrinology*, **48**(3), pp. R31–43.

,9      Pantziarka P, Sukhatme V, Bouche G, Meheus
        L and Sukhatme VP (2015) **Repurposing
        Drugs in Oncology (ReDO)-itraconazole as
        an              anti-cancer              agent.**
        *Ecancermedicalscience*, **9**, p. 521.

10      Pantziarka P, Bouche G, Meheus L, Sukhatme
        V and Sukhatme VP (2014) **Repurposing
        drugs in oncology (ReDO)-cimetidine as an
        anti-cancer agent.** *Ecancermedicalscience*, **8**,
        p. 485.

11      Kubecova M, Kolostova K, Pinterova D,
        Kacprzak G and Bobek V (2011) **Cimetidine:
        an anticancer drug?** *European journal of
        pharmaceutical sciences : official journal of
        the European Federation for Pharmaceutical
        Sciences*, **42**(5), pp. 439–44.

12      Deva S and Jameson M (2012) **Histamine
        type 2 receptor antagonists as adjuvant
        treatment for resected colorectal cancer.**
        *The Cochrane database of systematic reviews*,
        **8**(8), p. CD007814.

13      Pantziarka P, Bouche G, Meheus L, Sukhatme
        V and Sukhatme VP (2014) **Repurposing
        Drugs in Oncology (ReDO)-mebendazole as**

an anti-cancer agent. *Ecancermedicalscience*, **8**, p. 443.

14    Van Nuffel AM, Sukhatme V, Pantziarka P, Meheus L, et al. (2015) **Repurposing Drugs in Oncology (ReDO)-clarithromycin as an anti-cancer agent.** *Ecancermedicalscience*, **9**, p. 513.

15    Sukhatme V, Bouche G, Meheus L, Sukhatme VP and Pantziarka P (2015) **Repurposing Drugs in Oncology (ReDO)-nitroglycerin as an anti-cancer agent.** *Ecancermedicalscience*, **9**, p. 568.

16    Powe DG, Voss MJ, Zänker KS, Habashy HO, et al. (2010) **Beta-blocker drug therapy reduces secondary cancer formation in breast cancer and improves cancer specific survival.** *Oncotarget*, **1**(7), pp. 628–38.

17    Horowitz M, Neeman E, Sharon E and Ben-eliyahu S (2015) **Exploiting the critical perioperative period to improve long-term cancer outcomes.** *Nature Reviews Clinical Oncology*, pp. 1–14.

18    Benish M, Bartal I, Goldfarb Y, Levi B, et al. (2008) **Perioperative use of beta-blockers and COX-2 inhibitors may improve**

immune competence and reduce the risk of **tumor metastasis.** *Annals of surgical oncology*, **15**(7), pp. 2042–52.

19    Pasquier E, André N, Street J, Chougule A, et al. (2016) **Effective Management of Advanced Angiosarcoma by the Synergistic Combination of Propranolol and Vinblastine-based Metronomic Chemotherapy: A Bench to Bedside Study**. *EBioMedicine*.

20    Chae YK, Yousaf M, Malecek M-K, Carneiro B, et al. (2015) **Statins as anti-cancer therapy; Can we translate preclinical and epidemiologic data into clinical benefit?** *Discovery medicine*, **20**(112), pp. 413–27.

# For The Love of George

## Irene Kappes

George Pantziarka, an extraordinary little boy, is diagnosed with cancer on the day of his second birthday. For the next couple of years, he is mostly to be found zooming around hospital corridors playing games in between chemotherapy, radical surgery and radiotherapy.

George survives and grows up determined not to let cancer define him. But he is plunged once again into a life of hospital appointments and treatments when, at the age of fifteen, he develops skin cancer and then a tumour in his jaw. In the years that follow, his struggle for survival takes him from London to Frankfurt and then halfway across the world to China.

As he reports on Facebook, by the age of 17 he: *"...will have had: 3 different types of cancer, 17 operations, 13 scars, 22 different vitamins, 7 chemotherapy drugs, 3 very powerful anti-sickness drugs, 2 very powerful pain killers and one pretty f****d up genetic disorder."*

This is an account of one young man's love of life - a story of warmth, humour and the human condition.

George passed away on 25th April 20011. This is his story.

*ISBN-10: 1502741482     ISBN-13: 978-1502741486*